TAKE CONTROL
OF YOUR BLADDER...
AND YOUR LIFE.

the ACCIDENTAL SISTERHOOD

{ Unlock the Power of Your Secret Squeeze }

Raymond A. Bologna, M. D.
Urology
Female Pelvic Medicine
and Reconstructive Surgery

&

Jennifer Heisel Mangano, M. A., P. T.
Physical Therapist
Female Pelvic Floor Fitness

{ Take Control of Your Bladder ... and Your Life }

with

J. J. Rodgers

and Forewords by
Kristene E. Whitmore, M.D.
Susan Kellogg, Ph.D., C.R.N.P.

Pelvic Floor Health, LLC

Published in the United States by Pelvic Floor Health, LLC.

The Accidental Sisterhood™ is a registered trademark
of Pelvic Floor Health, LLC.

Library of Congress Control Number: 2006927848

ISBN-10: 0-9788717-0-7
ISBN-13: 978-0-9788717-0-3

Book designed by Keathley Advertising.

www.AccidentalSisterhood.com

Printed in the United States of America.

First printing: June, 2006
Second printing: April, 2007

{ Foreword to *The Accidental Sisterhood* }

by Kristene E. Whitmore, M.D.
Professor and Chair of Urology
and Female Pelvic Medicine and Reconstructive Surgery
Drexel University
Philadelphia, Pennsylvania

Allow me to recount a little history to explain where *The Accidental Sisterhood* is coming from and why I believe that it's an important contribution to women's health today. About 15 years ago, I co-authored the book *Overcoming Bladder Disorders*. We didn't discriminate; it covered the waterfront: men and women, incontinence, cystitis, interstitial cystitis, prostate problems, and bladder cancer. Although accessible and informative, it was a big book and, as I realize now, was ahead of its time. That's not to say that bladder problems weren't as prevalent then as now. Women's bladder problems as treatable – and preventable – issues just weren't on the radar for most practitioners, or even for women themselves. Going forward to now, today, that is no longer the case.

As a woman and a urologist – an unusual combination then, though not so now – I've devoted my practice to treating mostly women and helped to hone a new specialty: female pelvic medicine and reconstructive surgery. A woman's pelvic area is as vulnerable as it is vital. Pelvic floor disorders, especially as they involve the bladder, deserved a more dedicated and informed approach within urology. Recognizing this, I and others have worked to enlarge this focus on women's problems through research and advanced training. Fellowship programs are now providing this important focus for physicians throughout the country. And therein lies more history.

Dr. Bologna spent a year's fellowship working at my side at Graduate Hospital in Philadelphia. Now he has chosen to share his experience and concern with a broader audience: women who will pick up this book and discover that they don't have to put up with the problems that women have endured for ages. They'll find that they can choose to correct them, whether it's through surgery or conservative pelvic floor muscle therapy. They'll also find that bladder urgency, leaking urine inappropriately, and sexual dysfunctions related to the pelvic floor are preventable and treatable. This knowledge alone should be worth a great deal to every woman.

Since I published in 1990, there has been a rush to publish books and pamphlets for women about their bladder disorders. None, I think, approach the subject quite as comprehensively or as entertainingly as *The Accidental Sisterhood*. It is succinct and practical. You will learn, laugh, and, perhaps, shed a tear for all the tears you shouldn't have had to shed, but now I hope you will discover a better life.

I also hope the Pelvic Health Foundation will continue its mission of further educating women about women and that we can continue to work together on future projects.

The Pelvic Health Foundation may be the champion we've all been waiting for.

Kristene E. Whitmore, M.D.
Philadelphia, Pennsylvania
May 23, 2006

{ Foreword to *The Accidental Sisterhood* }

by Susan Kellogg, Ph.D., C.R.N.P.
Director: Sexual Medicine
The Pelvic & Sexual Health Institute
Philadelphia, Pennsylvania

For too many years, "accidental" loss of urine, loss of fecal matter, loss of ability to feel sensations during sex, loss of arousal, and loss of desire were considered just to be . . . well, accidental. Problems like these were considered by women (and unfortunately by many clinicians) to be "just one of those things that happen as we get older, . . ." inevitable, no big deal, a "normal" part of the aging process.

What *The Accidental Sisterhood* points out is that accidental losses are a big deal, they aren't inevitable and women can age with dignity, continence and a zest for sexual fulfillment! This book is the right book for a woman of any age who wishes to learn about her pelvic floor muscles and how they relate to good (or poor) control of the functions "down there."

As a practicing medical sexologist, it is one of my first priorities to acquaint my patients who have a female sexual dysfunction (more than 40 percent of women) with proper use of the muscles in the genital region and how these muscles can enhance arousal, sexual sensation, orgasm, and how weak muscles can detract from sexual satisfaction.

It was during his medical fellowship in Philadelphia that Dr. Bologna and I first met and discussed how important these muscles are for women, both in terms of urinary problems and sexual problems. I am thrilled that his work in this book can now reach a large number of women, many of whom had never had the privilege of an adequate pelvic floor muscle assessment nor had an adequate sexual history. Now women can read and learn about their bodies first hand and go on to assist the medical community in treating them in a holistic, state-of-the-art manner. *The Accidental Sisterhood* is the appropriate book at the appropriate time for the appropriate audience by the appropriate authors. Thanks to their expertise, the material is presented in a straightforward and easy-to-read fashion. The urologic and sexual wellness that may result will be . . . well, no accident!

Susan Kellogg, Ph.D, C.R.N.P.
Philadelphia, Pennsylvania
May 22, 2006

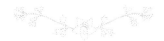

{ Acknowledgements }

Jeanette Geer of Keathley Advertising for her drive and commitment to get us, and keep us, on course.

Tom Keathley and his creative staff for their brilliant concepts for our book, our video, and our Web site, with special thanks to Jackie Bebenroth for her fine copyediting skills and insight, Doug Herberich for his designs, and Sara Myers for taking such good care of us.

Scott Chapski for his close reading of the text, for holding it to a high standard of consistency and clarity.

Our families for all the things they so richly and generously gave to us as we did our work for *The Accidental Sisterhood*: patience, love, and unquestioning support.

And especially to Isabella Bologna, Brooke Smith, Nicolette and Alex Mangano, who represent for us *every* daughter and granddaughter wherever they may be. That they may realize their full potential as healthy and confident young women, empowered by just one simple rule: know thyself.

As in *The Accidental Sisterhood*.

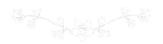

{ Note to Readers }

The information in *The Accidental Sisterhood* is
intended to help you improve the health and fitness
of your pelvic floor and should not be considered as
a substitute for the medical advice of a physician or
other health-care professional. Further, none of the
the information furnished in the text about medical
products and devices is an endorsement of them by
the authors or the publisher or of any claims made
for them by their manufacturers. It is always wise
to consult your own medical doctor or health-care
professional before embarking on any course of
treatment affecting your health and well-being.

CONTENTS

the
ACCIDENTAL
SISTERHOOD

Preface to *The Accidental Sisterhood*

{ The Untold Story of Untold Millions }

There's a story that women everywhere know, but which is rarely ever told. It takes place at a movie or at a mall, sometimes in a boardroom, and often in a bedroom. The setting can be anywhere. Only the plot never varies: the business or the moment at hand can't wait — and neither can your bladder.

And when the story is told, it often concludes with words like these: "I want to teach aerobics again. I want to play in the park with my children. I want to have sex with my husband and not worry that I'll have an urge to go, and when we do make love I want to feel something more in return. I want my life back."

Then, there's the other side of the story. Go into any one of the large drugstore chains and you'll find a sign above an aisle that says "Incontinence." There, right next to the menstrual products, are shelves of super-absorbent, pricey incontinence pads, liners, and briefs clearly and conveniently displayed for all who belong to . . . *The Accidental Sisterhood.*

Active, healthy women should not have to depend on these products, yet, judging by the size of the market for them, millions do.

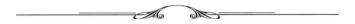

{ Nothing to Sneeze At }

Helping people hide their embarrassment is big business. Annual sales of adult incontinence pads and diapers run to about six billion dollars. Most of those who use these products – by a significant margin – are women. In their advertising, and to their credit, manufacturers of adult absorbent products do advise consumers to see a health-care professional about their bladder-control problems. Nevertheless, the open and candid way in which these products are now advertised, in print and on television, suggests that they are a woman's only solution to her problem, but, in fact, they are not.

The Accidental Sisterhood numbers 34 million American women . . . we think. It's probably more than that; the estimated numbers are all over the map. The National Institutes of Health report that 50 percent of all women have occasional urinary incontinence, with about 20 percent of women over the age of 75 experiencing daily urinary incontinence.[1]

Another study, funded by an international pharmaceutical

---

[1] *Medical Encyclopedia: Stress Incontinence.* National Institutes of Health, www.nlm.nih.gov/medlineplus/ency/article/000891.htm.

company and reported in *The New York Times*, found that 55 percent of women in their 80's are incontinent, and for women ages 30 to 39, 28 percent leak urine at least once a month.[2] Given these findings, it's anyone's guess what the absolute numbers are.

Why can't we be more precise than that? We can't because we don't know.

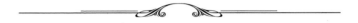

{ The Inconvenient Ones }

It's estimated that more than half of the elderly people in nursing homes are there because their families can't deal with their incontinence (both urinary and fecal). It's the number one reason for adult placement in nursing homes in the United States. No one should want to end her life wearing a diaper.

We don't know the full extent of female bladder-control problems for a couple of reasons. The social stigma attached to it is a painful reality for women who live every day with the mortifying possibility of wetting through their clothes, of having an odor, or of having to flee the dinner table for fear of leaking. Nor is it something they want to talk about with friends and family. Funny, isn't it? Women who wouldn't hesitate to bring up almost any other personal subject when with close friends would never mention their own bladder-control problems.

Many women – and men, as well – don't even tell health-

---

[2] "Enduring Incontinence In Silence," Science Times, *The New York Times*, October 25, 2005

care professionals because leaking urine is such a potent cultural taboo. *We know this because only one in 12 incontinent people sees a health-care professional for help.*[3] Either they fear that the problem wouldn't be taken seriously enough to warrant treatment (which is often the case), or they're in denial: "I'm too young to have this problem." "It happens only when I exercise." "I always leak a little when I have to go real bad. I didn't know I had a problem."

Not only do many people not want to talk about or recognize the problem, but according to another recent study reported in the *Times*, as many as two-thirds of them aren't doing anything to manage it except, perhaps, using absorbent pads.[4] Many women endure urinary incontinence for years before they mention it to health-care professionals.

The sad fact of the matter is that many women with bladder-control problems accept their fate. They believe, or have been led to believe, that it's a normal consequence of having a baby or two, of getting older, or for just being a woman.

Well, ladies, it's *not* your lot in life. It's not a natural consequence of having babies, of growing older, or of being a woman, and you *can* do something about it.

If you belong to *The Accidental Sisterhood*, it's safe to say you have great strength in numbers. But you have yet to flex your muscles to demand a greater level of concern for your problem.

---

[3] "Why Incontinence Need Not Be a Problem." www.pdrhealth.com, a service of Thomson Healthcare.

[4] *The New York Times.* Op. cit.

You shouldn't have to stay home and away from other people or near a bathroom because of the uncontrollable urge to urinate. You shouldn't have to fear wetting yourself when you laugh, sneeze, or exercise. You shouldn't have to avoid sexual intercourse because it's embarrassing, maybe uncomfortable, or it's gotten so you don't feel satisfied anymore. And you shouldn't have to worry that any of this may start happening to you sometime tomorrow or the day afterward. You can learn to flex your muscles, literally, to change your life, by yourself, for yourself.

The Accidental Sisterhood will help you understand what's wrong and how to make it right in a matter of a few weeks, or even sooner – and keep it that way for good.

Welcome to *The Accidental Sisterhood*
Raymond A. Bologna, M. D.
Jennifer Heisel Mangano, M. A., P. T.

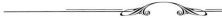

{ An Intimate Connection }
What does bladder control have to do with sex? A great deal. They both depend upon an innermost and intimate part of your body, one that most women know little about, yet that deeply influences the quality of their lives. It is, you will find, the central theme of **The Accidental Sisterhood.**

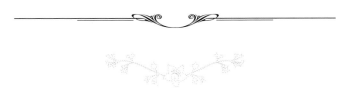

the
ACCIDENTAL SISTERHOOD

{ Introduction to Empowerment }

The Accidental Sisterhood is for women whose bladders give them no peace.

The Accidental Sisterhood is for women who leak urine when they laugh (or cough or sneeze or lift a growing child).

The Accidental Sisterhood is for sexually active women who wonder why sex isn't as satisfying as it used to be.

The Accidental Sisterhood is for every woman who, maybe like you, wants answers and a solution now for the problem she faces today, or may face tomorrow.

First, you should understand why you're having a problem: *The Accidental Sisterhood* will answer your questions. Second, The Accidental Sisterhood Progressive Plan will show you how to correct or prevent most problems – but not *every* problem. We will discuss other options for you, and, in the end, you'll have the information you need to know to make the right choice.

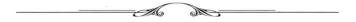

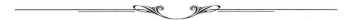

The Accidental Sisterhood shares more than a common experience. It goes deeper than that, to the core of every woman – her pelvic floor.

Maybe you have, or maybe you haven't, heard about it before, this "pelvic floor," it being down there and inside. Even if you have, its significance is still unknown to many women, and for some, it may be unmentionable.

Unknown, maybe. But unmentionable?

Not to us, and it certainly shouldn't be to you either. On the contrary, get set for empowerment. You are about to discover the pelvic floor in all of its anatomical glory. You will understand what it does for you, why it sometimes doesn't work as well as it should, and what you can do to make it fit and healthy again – and keep it that way. You'll learn practical techniques to harness the real and potential power of your pelvic floor and get it back in shape.

"I don't get it," you might say. "The pelvic floor? It sounds like a construction site." Well, in a way it is. The pelvic floor is important to all of us because it's a fundamental part of the conjoined and coordinated framework of bone and muscle that enables us to stand upright and make our way in the world as human beings.

The pelvic floor helps define us – and not insignificantly so – as male or as female.

It occupies the center of our gravity, holds sway over balance and posture, and is indispensable to the health and functioning of our sexual organs.

It's a complex arrangement of muscles, ligaments, and connective tissue that spans the pelvic opening between our legs.

It supports a woman's pelvic organs – the bladder, the vagina, the uterus, the rectum – and their pathways from her body.

It makes way for the birth of a child.

And it governs urinary and fecal continence.

But as vital as it is, a woman's pelvic floor is also vulnerable – susceptible to bladder overactivity, urinary incontinence, and sexual dysfunction: symptoms of an underlying disorder, signs that signify membership in The Accidental Sisterhood.

Treating pelvic floor disorder is the core of our practices in female urology and women's health physical therapy. We see women at all stages of the disorder, from a few drops of urine escaping with a little exercise to several soaked pads a day. We see women who can't leave their homes for fear of a sudden and uncontrollable urge to urinate. We see women who no longer achieve a satisfying sexual climax and who often avoid intercourse because of their bladder concerns. And at the extreme, when a pelvic organ loses the support of the pelvic floor, we see it protruding downward between the legs. These problems are correctable, and – for the millions of women who are unaware of what may be in store for them as they have their children and grow older – they are preventable. We repeat: *they are preventable.*

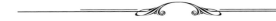

{ The Bump You Wish That Wasn't }
The condition characterized by the collapse of pelvic organs into the vagina and sometimes protruding out of the vagina is known as prolapse.

For a long time, correction meant surgery, except for a woman's sexual dysfunction. Even if she bravely raised that subject, nothing much was done for her in any event. But today we can do something for this and other problems through pelvic floor therapy, an alternative, conservative approach that has become the first line of treatment for pelvic floor disorder. As you'll soon see, its techniques are at the heart of our Accidental Sisterhood Progressive Plan – The Sisterhood Plan.

Until now, the authors' problem has been that we saw only one patient at a time. At that rate, we weren't making much of a dent in either problem: encouraging more women to seek therapy for a correctable problem or getting the word out to other women to prevent it. That's why we've made it our mission to reach out to you and every woman through this book, through other instructional media, and through our Web site, *www.AccidentalSisterhood.com.*

But even more critical than educating women about pelvic floor disorder is the need to offer a workable, non-surgical solution for it. It's what this book is all about. The Sisterhood Plan is a comprehensive approach to pelvic floor therapy that we've developed for our patients – and for you. It will, when you embrace it, make you better in ways that you may not have thought still possible. You can expect results in about four to eight weeks, and in some cases even sooner.

And so The Sisterhood Plan is for you if you live according to your bladder's time schedule, if you laugh and leak, if you only remember what sexual gratification used to be like, and you're among The Accidental Sisterhood who *know* they have a problem and simply won't accept it as your way of life.

And so The Sisterhood Plan is for you if you can't control your bladder, if going to the gym is out of the question, if you're finding that the feeling is not quite the way it used to be deep in the delta of Venus, and you're among The Accidental Sisterhood who'd rather *not think* about it but really know they *should.*

And so The Sisterhood Plan is for you if you're *not yet* counted among The Accidental Sisterhood . . . and you don't ever want to be.

Up ahead in this book you'll find what you need to know to stay dry and in control of your bladder and, once again, to savor sexual intimacy. Start down that path right now if you like. Go directly to **The Accidental Sisterhood Progessive Plan: Getting to Work**, and get to work. *But, please, you really should read the book all the way through.* You won't regret it. It won't take you long to find out what the problem is all about and how you, or your sister, your mother, your best friend, or even your daughter can change what shouldn't be any woman's fate. You need to know. They need to know.

{ Behold the Pelvis }

The Pelvic Floor . . . The Pelvic Organs . . . Down There . . .
The End of the Line

To understand the causes of urinary incontinence and sexual response disorders and why The Sisterhood Plan will help you, you ought to know something about the anatomy of the female pelvis. Careful, don't laugh. You'd be surprised at how many of our women patients harbor imprecise notions about how things are arranged down there. You may not find this section terrifically amusing, but you will find it factual. If you don't care to know all that much about your anatomy, skip it. If you just want to know a little something more about yourself, the illustrations and their descriptions will do that for you. At the very least, skim through the illustrations. This will give you a general understanding of the key muscle groups that make up the pelvic floor. It will increase your success rate when you start The Accidental Sisterhood Progressive Plan.

Okay? Still with us? The first thing you need to know is why you're built the way you are. That's because, to walk upright, as we do, we need a strong and durable framework of bones to rest upon the legs and to support the spine and the body around it. Behold the *pelvis*.

The human female pelvis is a remarkable structure. It is a large, as if sculptured, group of bones:

❀ Two flared, wing-like bones – the hipbones *(ilia)* – join together in front to create the pubic bone.
(See illustrations 1 & 2)

❀ The *sacrum*, a triangular bone made up of five fused vertebrae, and the *coccyx*, a small triangular bone at the base of the spinal column (the tailbone) form the back of the pelvis and anchor the spine, or vertebral column, to it. *(See illustrations 1 & 3)*

❀ The hipbones, pubic bone, sacrum and coccyx enclose the pelvic area and create the *pelvic cavity*, at the bottom of which is the *pelvic outlet*, the opening through which a child enters the world. *(See illustration 2)*

The pelvis may be remarkable, but it isn't perfect. Walking upright and having a pelvis big enough for a large-brained infant to fit through on her way into the world required a trade off. In most mammals that walk on all fours – including most primates – the weight of the abdominal and pelvic organs falls on the abdominal wall and the pubic bone. In humans, the weight funnels down upon a membrane of muscles and fibrous tissue about the thickness of a hand stretched across the inferior opening of the pelvic bowl. It is the *pelvic floor*.

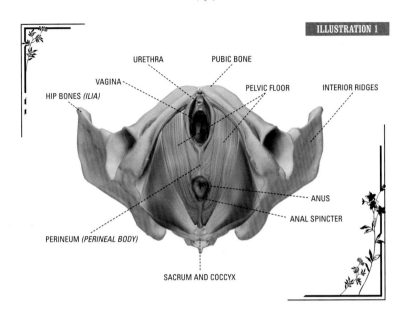

ILLUSTRATION 1

URETHRA
PUBIC BONE
VAGINA
PELVIC FLOOR
HIP BONES *(ILIA)*
INTERIOR RIDGES
ANUS
ANAL SPINCTER
PERINEUM *(PERINEAL BODY)*
SACRUM AND COCCYX

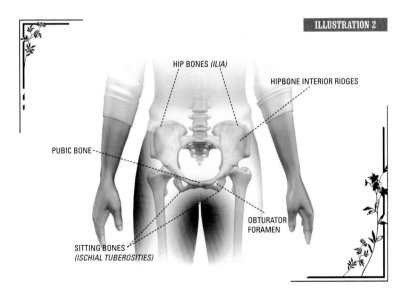

ILLUSTRATION 2

HIP BONES *(ILIA)*
HIPBONE INTERIOR RIDGES
PUBIC BONE
OBTURATOR FORAMEN
SITTING BONES *(ISCHIAL TUBEROSITIES)*

the
ACCIDENTAL SISTERHOOD

THE PELVIC FLOOR

Think of the pelvic floor as a hammock. The supporting "fabric" consists of two interlocking layers of muscle slung front to back from the pubic bone (in front) to the lower spine (*sacrum*) and the tailbone (*coccyx*) at the base of the spine (in back). *(See illustrations 3 & 4)* The layers of muscle are attached at the sides to the interior ridges (*ischial spines*) of the large hipbones (*ilia*) and the so-called sitting bones (*ischial tuberosities*), which protrude downward from each hipbone. *(See illustration 2)*

It's this hammock of muscle – the pelvic floor – that requires your attention. It's what you'll be learning to exercise and strengthen with The Sisterhood Plan. Even though you won't be able to "see" what you're doing, you'll soon "feel" it.

Each layer of the pelvic floor has a specific function:

❀ **The lower layer controls**. The lower layer of muscle is essentially horizontal and is sometimes referred to as the perineum. It covers the inferior opening of the pelvis – the pelvic outlet – and contributes significantly to the control of urination and to sexual pleasure. *(See illustration 4)*

❀ **The upper layer supports**. The upper layer of muscles is called the pelvic diaphragm and is shaped like a basin. It provides the main support to the pelvic organs and helps control the emptying of the bowel. *(See illustration 3)*

Thus, the muscles of the pelvic floor have four functions:

❀ To support the pelvic organs.

❀ To provide an elastic passageway for the birth of a child.

❀ To contribute to sphincter control and the elimination of wastes – the indispensable role that pelvic floor muscles play in helping you control your bladder and bowel.

❃ To enable and encourage reproduction through sexual intercourse and gratification.

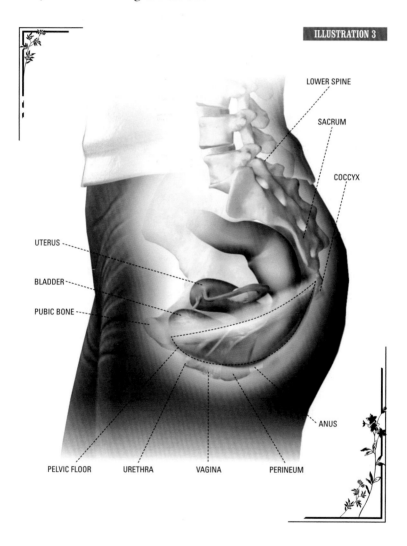

ILLUSTRATION 3

LOWER SPINE

SACRUM

COCCYX

UTERUS

BLADDER

PUBIC BONE

ANUS

PELVIC FLOOR   URETHRA   VAGINA   PERINEUM

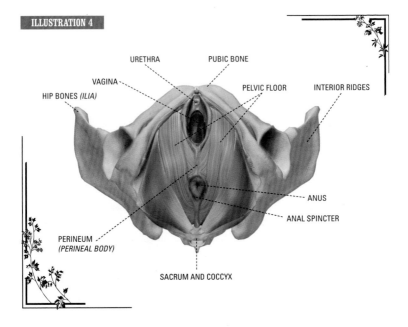

ILLUSTRATION 4

URETHRA   PUBIC BONE

VAGINA

HIP BONES *(ILIA)*   PELVIC FLOOR   INTERIOR RIDGES

ANUS

ANAL SPINCTER

PERINEUM
(PERINEAL BODY)

SACRUM AND COCCYX

To understand more about the muscles of the pelvic floor, you need to know more about muscles. Our bodies have two types of muscle groups – voluntary and involuntary. The muscles of the pelvic floor are, for the most part, voluntary. Of course, all muscles are controlled through the brain and central nervous system, but those that you can consciously control are known as *voluntary muscles*. Those that the brain controls without your conscious help are known as *involuntary muscles*.

The movements of your intestines and the contraction of your bladder are performed by involuntary (or smooth) muscles, which are controlled by your nervous system and seem to work automatically. When your rectum or bladder is full, the contractions of their involuntary muscles are felt as the urge to go to the bathroom.

{ Behold the Pelvis }

Voluntary (striated or long, striped) muscles are those that you can consciously contract and relax, or release, such as the large muscles of your arms and legs. These large muscles directly benefit from regular exercise. Like your arms and legs, the muscles of the pelvic floor, which are also striated or long muscles, benefit from regular exercise – and weaken if not exercised.

When your legs have grown weak, you may not be able to run or even walk. When you can't contract your pelvic floor muscles to help the anus and urethra maintain effective seals, the contractions of the bladder and bowel will overwhelm your ability to control them and you will leak.

In addition, when you can't contract the muscles around the vagina and hold the squeeze firmly around your partner's penis – the vaginal embrace – neither of you may enjoy the encounter quite as much as you should. When you have strong pelvic floor muscles, you'll find sexual intercourse more pleasurable for both you and your partner. You will both experience heightened sensation.

{ *When the Music Stops* }
Decreased sensitivity during sex is a problem for many women. We know this because patients have told us so. It's also made evident simply by virtue of the great number of lifestyle books and articles that are published about it. Unfortunately, aside from a few notable exceptions, most of
– continued on next page –

the
ACCIDENTAL SISTERHOOD

the authors either fail to fully understand the disorder or don't offer realistic solutions. It's also unfortunate that there is little to be learned from the medical literature, although that is changing. The success of sildenafil (Viagra®) and other drugs to treat male erectile dysfunction has stimulated a demand for sexual response drug therapies for women. Female sexual dysfunction is a multi-faceted problem that has social, psychological, and physical causes. Our focus is on correcting a specific physical cause that, once corrected, may contribute to a healthier emotional response. But whatever the cause of the problem, women are often left feeling needlessly guilty and inadequate because of it.

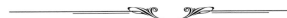

The pelvic floor has another special part to play in reproduction. It's what gives way when a child is pushed into the world and which may be injured while giving birth. It can also be injured in surgery, and it may grow thin (*atrophy*) and weaken with age. The pelvic floor, as we said, is vulnerable to many forces. But here's the good news: the pelvic floor can be repaired, strengthened, and preserved through The Sisterhood Plan.

In a healthy pelvic floor, the pelvic organs support each other and are supported in turn by the muscles and ligaments of the pelvic floor. For example, the uterus rests upon the bladder, which sits behind and slightly above the pubic bone. And the vagina is held in place from behind by the rectum. It is also anchored in place by the *perineal body*, a dense, fibrous membrane that spans the pelvic outlet between the vagina and the anus. *(See illustration 5)*

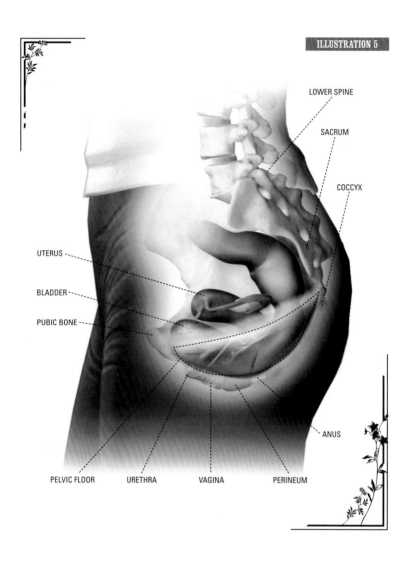

ILLUSTRATION 5

LOWER SPINE

SACRUM

COCCYX

UTERUS

BLADDER

PUBIC BONE

ANUS

PELVIC FLOOR   URETHRA   VAGINA   PERINEUM

The perineal body is at the center of the action. The Sisterhood Plan will require you to spend some quality time with this area. It plays an important structural role in the pelvic floor. It's where the supporting tendons and the muscles that span the pelvic outlet converge to form the perineum, or the lower layer of the pelvic floor (which we mentioned earlier). The muscles of the perineum weave around the perineal body to form two interlocking triangles – the urogenital triangle, in front, and the anal triangle, in back. The apexes *(the top points)* of these two muscle triangles meet at the perineal body at a point between the vagina and the anus. If you touch yourself there when you contract your pelvic floor muscles, what you feel pulling upwards is the perineal body.

Healthy pelvic floor muscles maintain a constant, resting tone, or tension, under the pelvic organs, until called into action –

- ❀ Contracting when you cough or sneeze to help the sphincters stay closed.
- ❀ Contracting when you want to suppress an urge to urinate.
- ❀ Relaxing when it's time to empty your bladder or bowel.
- ❀ Squeezing (contracting) during intercourse.

The pelvic floor functions much like the muscular *pulmonary diaphragm* that separates your abdominal and chest cavities and which, among other functions, controls your breathing. When you engage in aerobic exercise, you strengthen it. It's the same thing with the pelvic floor muscles: as you will see, when you exercise them, you will strengthen them and gain greater control.

THE PELVIC ORGANS

Three organs occupy the crowded space within a woman's lower pelvic cavity. Each organ belongs to a different system: *(See illustrations 6 & 7)*

* ❀ The uterus (the womb) – the reproductive system.

* ❀ The rectum (the last section of the large intestine) – the digestive system.

* ❀ The bladder (the muscular reservoir that collects urine excreted from the kidneys) – the urinary system.

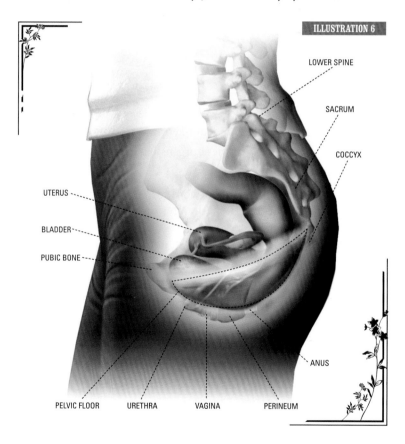

ILLUSTRATION 6

LOWER SPINE

SACRUM

COCCYX

UTERUS

BLADDER

PUBIC BONE

ANUS

PELVIC FLOOR   URETHRA   VAGINA   PERINEUM

ILLUSTRATION 7

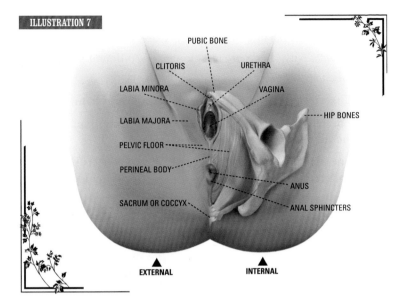

PUBIC BONE

CLITORIS

URETHRA

LABIA MINORA

VAGINA

LABIA MAJORA

HIP BONES

PELVIC FLOOR

PERINEAL BODY

ANUS

SACRUM OR COCCYX

ANAL SPHINCTERS

▲ EXTERNAL   ▲ INTERNAL

These organs are supported and kept in place above the legs by the pelvic floor. Each of these organs has a pathway from the body through the pelvic floor:

- ❀ The vagina, from the Latin word for "sheath," connects to the uterus at the *cervix* (the uterine portal) and serves a dual purpose:

  - ~ As a sexual organ and passageway for sperm to the uterus (unless blocked by a diaphragm or condom).

  - ~ As the birth canal and the channel to carry the monthly flow of blood and cellular debris from the uterus (*menses*).

- ❀ The anus, which connects to the rectum through the anal canal, carries fecal waste from the body.

- ❀ The urethra, which connects to the bladder, carries urine from the body.

DOWN THERE

The pelvic cavity is home to a woman's reproductive system. It's the sacred, almost magical, temple of fertilization, gestation, and birth. It contains and protects the uterus, and just above the uterus, the ovaries and fallopian tubes, which carry the ova to the uterus. If any place can be said to be "the center of life," this is it.

When a woman is not pregnant, her uterus is about the size of a plum and occupies a small space between the bladder and rectum. But in pregnancy, her uterus/womb becomes an exceptionally expandable organ of extraordinary strength, capable of sustained and powerful exertion during her labor to give birth to her child. It is this forceful expulsion of the child from the womb and through the pelvic outlet that often tears and weakens the muscles and tissues of her pelvic floor. Sometimes it damages the nerves that serve her bladder. And then one day, perhaps not too far off, she can't control an urge to urinate or may leak when she laughs.

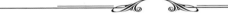

{ Helping Baby's Passage }

Not every woman's pelvic floor is injured when giving birth, but many are. To avoid injury, such as tearing the perineum as the child's head emerges, and to ease the passage of the infant through the birth canal, doctors will sometimes cut into the perineum layer to widen the birth canal – a procedure known as an **episiotomy.**

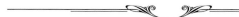

The pelvic cavity also makes room for the vagina where it rises, between the bladder and the rectum, to the uterus. Cylindrical in shape, it is about three and half inches long, extending from the *cervix* (the portal to the uterus), to the *vulva*, the collective term for the external female genitalia:

Both the vagina and the urethra open externally in the vulva and are enclosed by: *(see illustration 8)*

* ❋ The *labia majora*, the rounded folds of hair-bearing skin on either side of the vaginal vestibule, front to back.

* ❋ The *labia minora*, two thin, irregularly edged, inner folds of skin within the vestibule of the vagina that cover the vaginal and urethra openings and meet above the clitoris.

* ❋ The *clitoris*, a small, elongated erectile organ at the front of the vulva, with roots that extend deep into the pelvic floor.

ILLUSTRATION 8

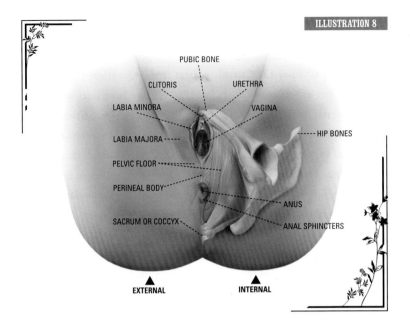

PUBIC BONE

CLITORIS

URETHRA

LABIA MINORA

VAGINA

LABIA MAJORA

HIP BONES

PELVIC FLOOR

PERINEAL BODY

ANUS

SACRUM OR COCCYX

ANAL SPHINCTERS

▲
EXTERNAL

▲
INTERNAL

The only function of the clitoris is sexual pleasure. Physical stimulation of the clitoris during sexual relations usually results in orgasm. Only somewhat like the penis, the clitoris becomes engorged with blood during sexual arousal, but very much *unlike* the penis, blood runs in and out of the clitoris, permitting successive multiple orgasms.

The lining of the vagina has two, thin layers of involuntary muscle:

* A superficial layer of muscle lies just beneath the inner vaginal surface, its fibers running the length of the vagina.

* Beneath the superficial layer is a sub-layer of muscle, its fibers encircling the vagina.

the
ACCIDENTAL SISTERHOOD

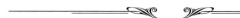

{ G-Spot Or Clitoris – That is the Question }
*In an article published in 1950 (*The International
Journal of Sexology, *February, 1950), Dr. Ernest
Gräfenberg reported that an area on the front, or anterior,
wall of the vagina along the "course of the urethra" is an
erotic zone and responds to stimulation by the finger. He
observed that during orgasm this area protrudes downwards
against the finger like a small cystocele, or bump. This
bump has since been referred to as the Gräfenberg spot, or
G-spot, but he makes no reference to its presence before
orgasm. Since then, the search has been on for the G-spot.
As it happens, a G-spot doesn't appear in all vaginas –
women are not all made exactly alike. The clitoris, however,
clearly exists and is a much larger and longer organ than
meets the eye; only the bud, or glans, is visible. The rest of
it rises up and out of sight into the perineum and divides,
like the letter Y, into two legs, or roots (*crura*), that extend
back, on either side of the urethra, to the vagina. One might
easily speculate that the G-spot phenomenon may be rooted
in the amazing and resourceful clitoris.*

The vagina does not have a *sphincter* (a ring of muscle),
although the muscular fibers of the lining are more developed
at the bottom third of the vagina. The tissues in this area of
the vagina are also rich in nerve endings and, according to
Dr. Elizabeth Gunther Stewart in her book, *The V Book,*

A Doctor's Guide to Complete Vulvovaginal Health, the tissues will swell around ("grasp") the penis during intercourse. What she is referring to is the *orgasmic platform* of the pelvic floor.[6]

The vaginal lining, or membrane, undergoes two marvelous and indispensable changes – one for sexual intercourse, the other for giving birth. The vagina opens during sexual intercourse and releases secretions to permit the penis to enter and move comfortably. During pregnancy, to ease the baby's passage, it becomes much more elastic. In preparation for the birth, the vaginal membrane stretches and folds in upon itself, like the pleats of an accordion, thus preventing all but superficial tearing to the vaginal walls of most healthy women as a child emerges.

Because the muscles in the lining of the vaginal membrane are not voluntary muscles, you can't consciously contract or relax them. When it's said that during intercourse a woman is squeezing her vagina to hold her partner's penis – the vaginal embrace – she is actually contracting the muscles of her pelvic floor. And it's the pulsating contractions of the pelvic floor muscles that are felt so intensely during orgasm. The stronger the muscles, the stronger the stimulation during intercourse and, usually, the stronger the orgasm. Sexual intercourse exercises the pelvic floor and is good for it. Orgasms are even better.

---

[6] *The V Book, A Doctor's Guide to Complete Vulvovaginal Health*, Stewart, E. G. and Spencer, P. Bantam Books, New York, 2002.

THE END OF THE LINE

Consider this the next time you finish a meal: everything you just ate is on its way through your digestive system. It starts in your mouth and ends at the pelvic floor. The digestive system's job is to extract nourishment and fluid from the things that you eat and drink as they move through the various stages of your system. Then, at the end of the line, it eliminates what's left over. That's the job of the rectum.

The rectum is the last section of the large intestine. It's located above the anus and at the back of the pelvic cavity behind the uterus and the vagina. The rectum expands to hold digestive waste, or *feces*. The walls of the rectum have two layers of involuntary muscle that contract to move fecal matter through the *anal canal* and from the body through the anus, the terminal orifice of the body's digestive system. But not until you let it happen. That's where two other muscles – *sphincters* – come in.

The sphincter muscles – an internal sphincter and an external sphincter – encircle the anus. The internal sphincter is, in effect, the anal orifice. It is smooth muscle and functions involuntarily (reflexively). The external sphincter surrounds the anal orifice and is incorporated within the pelvic floor. It's a voluntary muscle that can be contracted and relaxed at will. But it also gets help when needed. One of the muscles of the pelvic diaphragm loops around behind the external sphincter from the pubic bone and, when contracted, helps control the urge to evacuate.

To sum it up, emptying your bowel is a combination of voluntary and involuntary actions. In a resting state, the two anal sphincters, with help from the muscle loop supplied by the pelvic diaphragm, will keep the anal orifice closed. When the rectum is full, the two layers of muscles in its wall begin to move the contents toward the anal canal, and the internal sphincter relaxes. This is perceived as the urge to empty your bowel. Now, one of two things can happen: evacuation is immediately convenient, or it must be postponed. If it's convenient, you relax the external sphincter and the pelvic floor muscle that loops around it, and evacuation is accomplished.

If it isn't convenient, you will consciously contract the external sphincter surrounding the anus to suppress the urge. As the rectum continues to fill, the urge will return and will probably become stronger. This is when you need the muscle loop of the pelvic floor, as well. This muscle acts like a strap around the sphincter to pull it closed until it's convenient for you to evacuate. It's your back-up system.

Since fecal incontinence is not the problem we're dealing with here, in the following section we'll limit our discussion to the workings of the urinary system, and specifically, the lower urinary tract.

Nevertheless, it's important to understand that urinary incontinence and fecal incontinence are closely related problems. Urinary incontinence is the loss of normal control of the bladder. Fecal incontinence is the loss of normal control of the bowel.

In most cases of fecal incontinence, muscle damage is involved. In women, this damage commonly begins during childbirth. Chronic constipation aggravates the problem; severe and prolonged straining to empty the bowel can further damage the nerves and weaken the pelvic floor. Then, later in life, loose stool *(diarrhea)*, which is more difficult to control than formed stool, often causes the problem to show up.

In addition, diseases, surgery, and radiation therapy can reduce the elasticity of the rectum, which may shorten the time between the first sensation of having to go to the bathroom and the uncontrollable urge to have a bowel movement.

As with the symptoms of overactive bladder and urinary incontinence, it's important to seek careful medical advice. Only your health-care professional can provide the complete medical evaluation you need to learn the cause of the problem and identify a correct course of treatment. Once you have been evaluated and have no signs of cancer or other severe medical condition, pelvic floor therapy can help bowel control much like bladder control.

For more information, please turn to **Healthy Bowel Function** in the **Appendix**.

{ The Problem of Urinary Incontinence }

Holding It . . . Transient Factors . . . The Ninety-Nine Percent Sisterhood . . .
Underlying Issues of Urinary Incontinence . . . Just One More Thing

Urinary incontinence and bladder-control problems usually do not involve the kidneys. Located above the bladder in the back of the abdominal cavity, the kidneys (you're born with two of them) filter wastes, such as urea, from the blood. The kidneys combine the wastes with excess fluid to produce urine. The urine passes from the kidneys, a drop at a time through two tubes called *ureters*, and down to the bladder where it is stored until you urinate. When you urinate, you relax your pelvic floor muscles, which, in turn, signals the muscles that keep the urethra closed to relax and open. The bladder contracts, squeezing the urine out of the body through the urethra.

HOLDING IT

As with the anus, the muscles that keep the urethra closed are
called sphincters. The urethra has two sphincters:

● The *internal sphincter* is a ring of muscle within the urethra
  located up close to the bladder. It's normally closed, or
  contracted. It's an involuntary muscle, which means that it
  relaxes and opens reflexively in response to the contraction
  of the bladder muscle.

● The *external sphincter* surrounds the urethra nearer to its
  opening in the vagina. The external sphincter is incorporated
  as part of the lower layer of pelvic floor muscles and, unlike
  the internal sphincter, the external sphincter is a voluntary
  muscle. It's the muscle you can contract to help postpone
  urination, or relax when you wish to urinate (that is, you
  let it go). When you do, you signal the bladder to contract

and the internal sphincter to relax. This muscle also comes into play during sexual intercourse, as part of a layer of muscles that surrounds the vagina. A woman is able to contract this muscle layer to tighten the vagina, increasing the sensation for both partners.

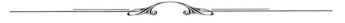

{ Bladder Control }

At the beginning of life, the bladder of an infant contracts automatically when a certain volume of urine is collected. As you learn to control urination, contraction of the bladder muscle (the detrusor muscle) is inhibited by a part of your brain (the cerebral cortex). It enables you to postpone urination until you are ready to urinate. By the same token, it also enables you to go even when you don't feel the need.

When the bladder has collected from eight to 10 ounces of urine, it activates nerves that give rise to the urge to urinate. An average bladder can hold as much as 20 ounces, but it doesn't wait until it's completely full before it lets you know that you need to go. It gives you a little wiggle room.

However, when you feel the urge to go, if you're not at a place where you can go to the bathroom just yet, you override the bladder's signal and keep the sphincters closed. As the bladder continues to fill, the urge to urinate becomes stronger. You can delay it only up to a point, at which time urination becomes unavoidable.

Thus, the business of normal urination is a coordinated involuntary and voluntary action. When your bladder is full, it lets you know that it's time to go by beginning to contract. This is felt as the urge to urinate. If a toilet isn't handy, you let it know "not yet" by contracting your pelvic floor muscles and suppressing the urge. When you do this, here's what happens: the urethral sphincter tightens up, the bladder muscle stops contracting, and the urge subsides. Then, when you're ready to go, here's what happens: you relax your pelvic floor muscles, the bladder muscle responds by contracting (as you might squeeze a rubber balloon), the urethra sphincter relaxes and opens, and urine is expelled.

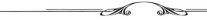

{ *How Often is Normal?* }
Normally, people need to urinate every three to four hours. Abnormally, in cases of overactive bladder, the urge to go can be felt every 30 minutes or so.

Urinary incontinence is a symptom that something isn't working right with your body. The exact causes are unclear. We know that all women are made a little differently; the strength of the support tissues of the pelvic floor varies from woman to woman.

Pregnancy often causes damage to the pelvic floor muscles and nerves. The added weight of the baby and the mother's womb can stretch the pelvic floor muscles and lead to incontinence after delivery, even if she delivers by caesarian section.

Pelvic surgery can weaken the pelvic floor muscles and interfere with nerves controlling the bladder. The constant pounding from training for and running a marathon won't help the cause, either. In time, the damage done by any or all of these stresses on the pelvic floor may result in incontinence.

❀ Lilly's Story ❀

I was the girl at the slumber parties who laughed so hard she peed her pants. That should've been my first warning. But I grew up knowing very little about bladder problems. My mother had leakage issues, but it didn't mean it would happen to me, ... right? Wrong. After I had my first baby, I was in serious trouble. I couldn't leave the house without thinking about protective measures. I couldn't hurry across the street from the parking lot to my office without leaking. I love to go dancing, and what should've been fun always turned into a strategic escape plan halfway through the evening. I was 34 the last time this happened to me. As we left, my husband turned to me and said, "You can't go on living like this." I didn't think he knew. I didn't want anybody to know.

TRANSIENT FACTORS

From time to time, it's not unusual for women to experience more frequent urges to urinate or leak under certain circumstances. Urinary incontinence may appear as a result of certain short-term, or transient, factors that have little if anything to do with the pelvic floor. Transient incontinence may occur suddenly and just as quickly disappear if certain offending substances are avoided or infections are cured. For example:

❈ *Medications.* They include diuretics, analgesics, sedatives, antihistamines, decongestants, and antidepressants. Please refer to the **Appendix** for a detailed list. If a prescribed medicine or over-the-counter remedy is the cause, the problem will diminish or disappear when the drug is discontinued or a substitute is prescribed. But be sure to see your health-care professional before you discontinue any prescription medication.

❈ *Infections.* Inflammations of the bladder, urethra, and vagina can also cause urinary incontinence. Often caused by a microbial *(bacterial)* infection, these issues are easily treated with antibiotics. Once treated, the incontinence clears up. *Important: If you see blood in your urine or have pain when you urinate, you need to contact your doctor immediately.*

Whatever the external factor is, once it's eliminated by other medical means, the transient urinary incontinence usually goes away.

In any treatment plan, it's important to eliminate any transient factor first. *We can't stress enough the importance of discussing a bladder-control problem with your health-care professional.* Only by getting to the bottom of the problem can you begin to treat it effectively. And as we explicitly maintained at the outset, urinary incontinence is a very, very treatable problem. If you're reading this book before you see a health-care professional, you're ahead of the game. You can go to your first appointment with informed questions and know what to expect during an examination. (For detailed descriptions of the kinds of tests you might encounter, see **Getting to the Bottom of Your Problem – A Guide to Diagnosis**.)

THE NINETY-NINE PERCENT SISTERHOOD

The most common types of incontinence often come on gradually, usually worsen over time, and primarily involve the functions of a woman's lower urinary tract. These functions include:

* Storing urine in the bladder.
* Keeping the urethra closed.
* Squeezing urine through the urethra and out of the body.

In the earlier sections on the anatomy of the pelvic floor, you learned that a woman's lower urinary tract is a complex mechanism that involves a number of cooperating body parts: the brain and pelvic nerves, the bladder muscle, the urethra, and the muscles and ligaments of the pelvic floor. When this complex mechanism is out of whack, 99 percent of the time the problem will be the most common types of incontinence. They are overactive bladder, stress urinary incontinence, or a mixture of both conditions – simply called mixed urinary incontinence.

If you have a problem, there's a good chance that you'll find your symptoms below:

Overactive bladder is a bladder storage problem in which the bladder contracts suddenly and inappropriately. You feel it as a frequent and overpowering urge to go to the bathroom, night and day, followed by a powerful and uncontrollable bladder contraction. If the muscles that keep your urethra closed are weak, you won't make it to the bathroom in time. This is overactive bladder-*wet* (also called urge urinary incontinence). If your pelvic muscles are fit, you normally will get there in time. This is overactive bladder-*dry* (or, simply put, just urgency).

Stress urinary incontinence is also a bladder storage problem in which the muscles that normally stop the flow of urine are too weak to stop it when pressure is exerted on the bladder from the abdomen above. This causes you to leak urine as you stand up, or get out of a car, lift a heavy object, exercise, cough, sneeze, or laugh. Any action that creates downward pressure on the bladder and urethra or increases intra-abdominal pressure can cause you to leak urine. Some of you will remember your baby kicking your bladder when you were pregnant and what sometimes happened: you leaked.

In *mixed urinary incontinence*, not only do you leak when you lift, but you never want to find yourself where you can't find a bathroom. You have symptoms of both an overactive bladder and stress urinary incontinence.

Overactive bladder tends to appear later in life; its incidence increases with age and often worsens after menopause. Whereas many women first experience stress urinary incontinence in their younger years, surprised, at first, by leaking during an aerobics class or as they lift their toddlers.

The muscles of the pelvic floor have several jobs to do to keep you dry – on a battleground of countervailing forces:

- To maintain a constant, or resting tone, under the pelvic floor organs and keep them up where they belong.
- To tighten around the urethra as the urge to go to the bathroom increases.
- To contract quickly and firmly just as you start to laugh or cough or sneeze.

You also need to have the following things working for you:

- *A cooperative bladder.* It must store urine easily, like a well–used balloon.
- *A healthy bladder.* It shouldn't try to squeeze urine out at the wrong time.
- *A urethra that closes tightly.* The urethral sphincter, as well as your pelvic floor muscles, must form a tight seal when you laugh, cough, sneeze, stand up, or lift a heavy object.
- *A stable backboard for the bladder and urethra.* The ligaments that stabilize the bladder and the pelvic muscle around the urethra have to work together to keep the urethra closed.

A weak pelvic floor is not an indication of ill health; perfectly healthy women, both those who have and those who have not given birth, find that their pelvic floor muscles fail them as well. In fact, there are plenty of active, athletic women who are fit in every way except for their pelvic floors. No woman should consider herself immune.

{ Sisterhood Scenarios }

Putting it as simply and directly as we can, the problem of incontinence presents a number of possible scenarios. Consider the following:

❀ *What if your pelvic floor loses its tone and sags, and the organs and the complex urinary system sag with it? You are at risk for urinary incontinence.*

❀ *What if the angle between your bladder and urethra changes, and what if the sag puts a crimp in the urethra so that its sphincter can't close completely without the firm support it needs from the weakened pelvic floor muscles? What happens then if you cough hard? You will leak.*

❀ *What if trauma, childbirth, or disease has damaged the nerves of your bladder and the urethral sphincter, and your pelvic floor muscles have sagged, and your bladder contracts suddenly (as it often does)? And what if you're nowhere near a bathroom? You almost certainly will leak.*

❀ *What if you have an almost constant urge to go, your urethral sphincter can't close completely, and you can't contract weak pelvic floor muscles? And what if you cough, or laugh, or do whatever you do in the course of your active daily life? Don't ask.*

If you find yourself in any of these scenarios, the likely result will be ... well, an accident.

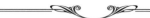

UNDERLYING ISSUES OF URINARY INCONTINENCE

Although we've already discussed a number of causes of urinary incontinence, there's still a need to address other issues often underlying or contributing to the disorder. Some are physiological; some are behavioral. Some you can control, some you can't.

For instance, consider the following issues:

* *Constipation.* Many patients we see for urinary incontinence report chronic constipation. The problems are often related to the fact that there's only so much room in the pelvic area. If your bowel is full of stool, the bladder has no place to go. A small amount of urine makes the bladder uncomfortably full, and you will often feel great urgency to urinate. Because of the closeness of the bowel to the bladder, the stool can actually irritate the bladder. In addition, straining at stool creates heavy pressure upon the pelvic floor and, over time, weakens the muscles' ability to support the pelvic organs.

* *Family history.* There is probably a genetic component to female urinary incontinence. The question remains: does it run in families and, if so, in what way? In all likelihood, it does. In some families the muscles of the pelvic floor may be prone to atrophy or weaken with age, or be such that they are unable to recover from the stretching they undergo during pregnancy or a vaginal delivery.

* *Disease.* Insofar as the bladder is concerned, diabetes and certain neurological disorders, such as multiple sclerosis (MS) and Parkinson's disease, are implicated in overactive bladder. A failure of the bladder to contract properly can also follow a stroke.

{ *Diseases Affecting Bladder Control* }

❀ *Diabetes can be any of several metabolic disorders marked by excessive discharge of urine and persistent thirst.*

❀ *MS is a chronic degenerative disease of the central nervous system. It causes a gradual destruction of the tissue (myelin) that covers nerve fibers in patches throughout the brain or spinal cord or both. The damage interferes with the nerve pathways and causes muscular weakness, loss of coordination, and speech and visual disturbances. The disease occurs chiefly in young adults and is thought to be caused by a defect in the immune system that may be of genetic or viral origin.*

❀ *Parkinson's disease is a progressive nervous disease occurring most often after the age of 50. It's associated with the destruction of brain cells that produce dopamine (a neural transmitter) and is characterized by muscular tremor, slowing of movement, partial facial paralysis, peculiarity of gait and posture, and weakness.*

❀ *A stroke, also called a cerebrovascular accident, is a sudden loss of brain function caused by a blockage or rupture of a blood vessel to the brain. It's characterized by loss of muscular control, diminution or loss of sensation or consciousness, dizziness, slurred speech, or other symptoms that vary with the extent and severity of the damage to the brain.*

❀ *Physical mobility.* Incapacitating conditions, such as arthritis, while not directly affecting the bladder or the pelvic floor muscles, are a major factor in urinary incontinence. A disabled person trying to get to a bathroom can take too long to get there even with a normal bladder. Functional urinary incontinence (as this is known) sends many elderly people to long-term care facilities, even though their urinary systems are working fine.

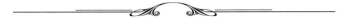

{ *When Disability is the Problem* }

The cause of functional incontinence is physical immobility or mental impairment. While their urinary systems may be working fine, the muscles and joints of elderly people may not be. Physical therapy can help improve their mobility, and pelvic floor therapy can help them control their urge to urinate until someone can help them to a bathroom. Then there are other people with dementia or impaired memory who can't recognize the physical signals that they must urinate. While their disabilities make them difficult to treat, they are treatable. Whatever the approach to treatment, it requires a team effort by their caregivers to preserve and restore their dignity.

❀ *Obesity.* Obesity has been found to be more common in incontinent women than in continent women. Studies report a significant correlation between high body-mass index and urinary incontinence. It suggests that greater intra-abdominal pressures overwhelm a woman's ability to control her urine flow. Our first objective is to make the patient dry by whatever means work best for her. This may include encouraging her to seek a weight-loss program and to add any form of exercise she sees fit to follow. In many cases, we are able to correct the incontinence so they feel comfortable exercising.

* *Hormones.* Estrogen depletion in postmenopausal women may adversely affect the bladder and urethra, which are known to be rich in estrogen receptors. The depletion causes tissues within the bladder, urethra, and vaginal area to atrophy (thin out) and become easily irritated. Support of the urethra and bladder can be compromised. We are mindful that estrogen replacement therapy is controversial. However, we often place our patients on vaginal estrogens for their local effect. Please consult your health-care professional for more information.

* *Fluid intake.* The popular (and mistaken) notion that one must drink at least eight eight-ounce glasses of water a day, in addition to all of the other fluids – coffee, iced tea, juice, sodas – that one might otherwise consume, may be just too much for any bladder to handle. Hence, excessive fluid intake may be mistaken for – or aggravate – an overactive bladder.

But make no mistake about it; it is equally important to drink an adequate amount of fluid every day. Too many women report that they do not drink enough fluids to maintain healthy bladder and bowel habits because they're afraid they might leak. Not getting enough fluid, however, can decrease the amount of urine the bladder can store and produce a more concentrated urine, which may lead to inappropriate bladder contractions, infections, and, hence, more leaks. Low fluid intake can also aggravate constipation.

So, listen up, please. Depending on your level of activity, or the heat and humidity of the day, we recommend that you take in at least six to eight eight-ounce glasses of non-irritating fluids every day. We'll discuss non-irritating fluids later.

{ *Let Thirst Be Your Guide – But Hold The Salt and Pass The Bananas* }

The Food and Nutrition Board of the Institute of Medicine reported in 2004 that the vast majority of healthy people adequately meet their daily hydration needs by letting thirst be their guide. The report did not specify exact requirements for water, but set general recommendations for women at 91 ounces of total water – from all beverages and foods – each day. For men, the amount was 125 ounces every day.

The report stated that about 80 percent of a person's total water intake comes from drinking water and beverages and the remaining 20 percent comes from food. For a woman, this comes to about nine eight-ounce glasses of a water-bearing liquid every day, which is one more than the minimum that we recommend.

Prolonged physical activity and heat exposure will increase water losses and, therefore, may raise daily fluid needs. The report cautions that drinking excessive amounts of fluid can be life threatening.

The report also calls attention to the importance of proper amounts of sodium chloride (table salt) and potassium in our diets. People, it points out, generally get too much salt and not enough potassium. Excessive salt intake contributes to high blood pressure and aggravates other diseases. Consuming about five grams of potassium (from bananas, for example, or a vitamin supplement) every day helps to lower blood pressure, blunts the effects of salt, and reduces the risk of kidney stones and bone loss. American women get only about half of the potassium they need every day.[7]

[7] "Dietary Reference Intakes: Water, Potassium, Sodium Chloride, and Sulfate," Food and Nutrition Board, Institute of Medicine of the National Academies, www.iom.edu.

* *Potty training.* Remember being told by your mom to make sure you went to the bathroom before you left the house, and to make sure that you never missed any opportunity to use the bathroom even if you didn't have to go? Maybe mom even ran water to help you go, or she made you sit there until you did. In some families, maintaining an empty bladder, like cleanliness, is next to godliness. That's bad news for you and all of the girls out there. And that's why some adult bladders need re-education. You should not have to go more than once every two to five hours. You should be able to make it to the grocery store and back.

* *Holding it.* The other side of the potty-training coin is not going when you should, an all-too-common habit for many women. Over time, women who hold their water for many hours at a stretch will find it difficult to empty their bladders and will often leak urine, as in overflow urinary incontinence. This problem is usually self-inflicted from too many years of "holding it." For whatever reason – too busy to take the time, never any place to go (no plumbing in sight or a toilet you just won't sit on) – you've trained your bladder to forget how to relax. The Sisterhood Plan will help you bring it back in line.

If being incontinent isn't bad enough, sometimes there's that egg-sized bulge some women find inside their vaginas. If their incontinence isn't enough to get them in to see a health-care professional, this'll do it – and it should. In short, the problem usually begins when their pelvic floor muscles literally let them down.

What they've found is a *pelvic organ prolapse.* It's another consequence of a weakened or damaged pelvic floor. As the pelvic floor muscles and ligaments holding the organs in place weaken, the bladder – or the uterus or the rectum – may begin to bulge down into the vagina creating this hernia-like condition.

Over time, if not treated, a prolapsed organ may descend into the vagina and literally turn the vagina inside out like a sock. You should see your health-care professional long before this happens. (See **Correcting Prolapse**.)

❈ Anna's Story ❈

A few years before my husband and I retired, I felt some vaginal pressure. My primary care doctor noticed a small bump in my vagina. He said it was the bladder pressing against the vagina. I had tried Kegel exercises when I was younger. I did them again for a while, and it helped to ease the pressure. But right after we retired, my husband got sick, and I took on the job of caring for him as he recovered. Just before he got back on his feet again, I was helping him out of the bathtub when something popped down inside me, and the pressure in my vagina became uncomfortable. When we resumed intercourse, there was something in the way. My gynecologist said that it was a cystocele: my bladder had lost the support it needed and was bulging down into my vagina. It was, in short, a prolapsed organ. It made me feel vulnerable. I'm 66 now, and I had looked forward to retiring. We both enjoy golf and travel – what we always planned to do when we could. Now, I don't know. I just don't feel like doing the things I did before.

The Sisterhood Plan is not meant to cure a urinary tract infection or correct a situation that clearly requires surgery. But it does improve most cases of urinary incontinence and bladder control, and can help with some of the conditions we've just described. What's more, its contribution to sexual response and pleasure for a woman can't be understated. In all respects, we believe that a stronger pelvic floor can show you the way to a stronger sense of yourself.

JUST ONE MORE THING

Lest we forget, perhaps you've noticed that we haven't mentioned male urinary incontinence. Well, what about the men in your lives? How do they figure in all of this? Men with prostate troubles will have difficulty urinating. And at a certain age, men and women have similar bladder-control problems almost in equal number. But our immediate concern is women. Throughout their lives, urinary incontinence strikes many more women than men. Part of the reason for this is how each sex is made. Just in case you never noticed, a man's pelvic floor has two orifices: for the urethra, which runs through the prostate gland and the length of the penis, and the anus. A woman's pelvic floor has, as of course you most certainly now know, three orifices: the urethra, the anus, and the vagina.

A woman's urethra, the tube through which urine is expelled from the bladder, is about an inch and a half long and, with menopause, may tend to shorten. A man's urethra is obviously longer. All other things being equal, the shorter the urethra the more likely the leak and the susceptibility to infection.

A woman's pelvic floor is more flexible than a man's, to allow for the passage of an infant through the birth canal. In and of itself, this flexibility predisposes women to the weakening of the pelvic floor. That is why the core of pelvic floor therapy concentrates on strengthening the muscles of the pelvic floor.

As you are about to embark on a new path to pelvic floor health, it's important to be mindful of the fact that, on the whole, many, many more women suffer from pelvic floor disorders than men do. If not you, then someone you know does; it's that prevalent. What's more, despite increasing attention to this problem, it's still largely unappreciated by the medical community due to a previous lack of treatment options. So it's about time that health-care professionals and physical therapists alike did something about it – just for women. A discussion of the problem of male urinary incontinence must wait for another time. This is for you. The Sisterhood Plan is about empowering women to make a difference in their own lives. And when they do, their men will surely feel the difference.

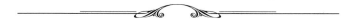

{ At-A-Glance Symptoms of Urinary Incontinence }
~ Most Common and Not-So Common ~

Here are the symptoms of the three most common types of urinary incontinence – overactive bladder–wet (urge urinary incontinence), stress urinary incontinence, and mixed urinary incontinence – and other not-so–common types of urinary incontinence.

– continued on next page –

the
ACCIDENTAL SISTERHOOD

Overactive Bladder–Wet

❋ *You frequently have a strong, sudden urge to urinate.*

❋ *You regularly go the bathroom eight or more times during a 24-hour period.*

❋ *You get up two or more times during the night to go to the bathroom.*

❋ *You leak on the way to a toilet.*

❋ *You leak all of a sudden for no good reason, just standing on the street talking to a friend or sitting in a movie.*

❋ *You never pass up a bathroom "just in case" you might need one later.*

❋ *You limit the amount of fluid you drink so there's less urine to leak.*

❋ *You come home from the grocery store and – "key in the lock" – it's your cue to make a dash for the bathroom. (We've heard that some patients leave their doors unlocked, so fumbling with a key in a lock won't slow them down.)*

(If you can usually keep from wetting yourself on the way to the bathroom, you can call your symptoms overactive bladder-dry.)

Stress Urinary Incontinence

❋ *You lose urine when you're doing physical activities, such as exercising or lifting heavy objects.*

❋ *You sometimes have a slight loss of urine (even if it's only a drop or two) when you laugh, sneeze, or cough.*

❋ *You can't sit down or stand up without wetting yourself.*

Mixed Urinary Incontinence

    ❋ *You experience most or all of the symptoms of overactive bladder–wet and stress urinary incontinence.*

Then, just in case you don't recognize your symptoms so far, here are symptoms of other, far less common forms of urinary incontinence:

Overflow Urinary Incontinence

    ❋ *You are unaware that you periodically leak small amounts of urine until you feel your pad is wet.*

    ❋ *You feel no urge to urinate, even though your bladder may be full.*

    ❋ *You can't completely empty your bladder or make it contract to expel urine.*

Functional Urinary Incontinence

    ❋ *You have a problem recognizing the signals that you need to urinate.*

    ❋ *You are physically unable to reach a bathroom in time.*

Continuous (Total) Urinary Incontinence

    ❋ *You have no control of urine flow, which leaks continuously into the vagina, a rare condition possibly caused by a hole in the bladder (a fistula) or an injury to the urethra.*

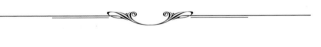

{ Getting to Work }

Introduction to a New Day ... How The Sisterhood Plan Works for You ...
Dr. Kegel's Legacy ... Don't Stop When You're Ahead

INTRODUCTION TO A NEW DAY

If you've stayed with us from page one, you've reached the point where you've learned all you need – or may want – to know about the Problem. From this point on, you'll find the Solution. If you follow The Sisterhood Plan, we believe you will improve the quality of your life.

In the opening pages of this book we wrote that many women do not seek help for overactive bladder and urinary incontinence. Our goal is to change that fact: that instead of ignoring the first signs of bladder instability and incontinence, women will choose to do something about it. Their first choice should be to see a health-care professional. *Ninety-nine percent of those who tell a health-care professional about their problem improve their quality of life.*

Once the possibility of infection or drug side effect is ruled out and no condition exists that requires immediate surgical repair or other invasive treatment, a patient can choose pelvic floor therapy. And those who do will benefit.

What's more, many patients who might elect to have surgery can avoid it with pelvic floor therapy. Of those women who choose pelvic floor therapy, a significant percentage of them – as high as 50 percent in some cases – ultimately avoid surgery. Furthermore, our experience suggests that women who start off with pelvic floor therapy and later go on to have surgery often recover better after surgery. If this sounds encouraging, it is. On the other hand, however, some women choose surgery over therapy; they want a quick fix. And it's their right to do so.

Invasive testing is rarely required before initiating conservative therapy. Conservative therapy, such as we set forth here, is safe and effective and should be considered as the first line of treatment for most patients.

An initial evaluation by your health-care professional should include, at a minimum, an assessment of the symptoms, a physical examination, including a pelvic exam, and a urinalysis to check for blood and infection. The purpose of this initial evaluation is to separate uncomplicated urinary incontinence – overactive bladder-wet, stress and mixed urinary incontinence – from complicated conditions that require further clinical assessment. Complicated conditions would include urinary fistula, pain, blood in the urine, significant pelvic organ prolapse, recurring urinary tract infections, and persistent incontinence after pelvic surgery or irradiation. (See **Getting to the Bottom of Your Problem – A Guide to Diagnosis** for the types of diagnostic tests used.)

Based on a preliminary diagnosis of your condition as uncomplicated overactive bladder-wet, stress, or mixed urinary incontinence, you should expect to begin a conservative treatment of eight to 12 weeks of pelvic floor therapy.

Conservative therapy is effective for the motivated patient. If that's you, you're already on your way. But even then, some patients need additional help to get them started. This help is available in the forms of biofeedback (to confirm that you're exercising the correct muscles), low-level electrical stimulation to activate the pelvic floor muscles, and exercising with progressive vaginal weights. More on all of this later.

As we've pointed out, it's not uncommon for some women to elect surgery over pelvic floor therapy. If you want to know more about the types of surgery used to correct the most common forms of incontinence, you'll find the information in **Surgery and Other Options for Overactive Bladder, Stress Urinary Incontinence, and Prolapse**.

HOW THE SISTERHOOD PLAN WORKS FOR YOU

Most of our patients and millions of women who have not sought treatment for the most common types of urinary incontinence and bladder-control problems stand to benefit from a conservative, non-surgical preventive and restorative approach to getting and staying dry.

the
ACCIDENTAL SISTERHOOD

If you choose our approach, you will work with us to begin to practice good pelvic floor health through a program of pelvic awareness and progressive strength-building exercises. In addition, practicing good bladder health and habits are also essential parts of The Sisterhood Plan.

The Sisterhood Plan works for you in three, interdependent ways:

* Bladder Training – Exercising mind over bladder.
* Progressive Pelvic Floor Exercises – Developing pelvic floor awareness and strength.
* Behavior Modification – Identifying personal habits and the things in your diet that may be at the root of your problem.

The objective of The Sisterhood Plan is to preserve and restore the health of a woman's pelvic floor. The three steps of The Sisterhood Plan – Bladder Training, Progressive Pelvic Floor Exercises, and Behavior Modification – are intended to be done together. You progress along three parallel paths, each advancing and enhancing your progress as you go.

Bladder Training – breaking old habits. Damage or disease can cause your bladder to contract urgently and involuntarily. But often, it "learns" to contract out of sheer habit. If you're like many women, you've spent most of your life unconsciously teaching your bladder never to pass up an opportunity to go, whether you really have to or not. Now you find that it doesn't take much to trigger the urge. Cues like running water, getting in the shower, or seeing a toilet will trigger the urge. You can break this old habit, as you will soon learn.

Progressive Pelvic Floor Exercises — re-building what you can't see.
Progressive Pelvic Floor Exercises can be challenging because you can't
actually see the results of your efforts. But you will soon begin to feel
the results — improved bladder control and sexual response — which are
the lifetime benefits of staying with the program for the long term.

Behavior Modification — changing your way of living. Getting rid
of the things in your life that undermine pelvic floor health will
earn you great rewards as you begin to strengthen the muscles
you can't see and re-educate a bladder you can't control.
Behavior Modification is all about making positive choices like
watching your diet, quitting smoking, and getting more exercise.
In many instances, Behavior Modification alone can alleviate
your symptoms of urinary incontinence.

❀ How It Got Better for Betsy ❀

I talked with Dr. Bologna about my frequent urges and
sudden losses of control. He started me on The
Sisterhood Plan. The Behavior Modification part was
key for me. The first thing I noticed was that coffee
made my urgency symptoms worse, and if I drank more
water, I didn't feel the need to go as often. Within two
weeks, my urgency and frequency improved. In the
meantime, I committed to my pelvic floor exercises. In
just one month, my husband noticed a difference, if you
know what I mean. And yes . . . it's better for me, too.
But that's not all; when I jog, I stay dry all the way.

DR. KEGEL'S LEGACY

Behavior Modification and Bladder Training are like the two ends of a bridge that spans the gap between pelvic floor disorder and pelvic floor health. But you can't get to the other side without the Progressive Pelvic Floor Exercises. The core of pelvic floor therapy is proper exercise. Most women have probably never heard about pelvic floor therapy. But many have heard about – and maybe tried – Kegels.

Suggested more than 70 years ago by Dr. Joshua Davies, a New York physician, the idea of exercising the pelvic floor as a remedy for incontinence floated around in the backwaters of medicine for many years. In the 1950s, Dr. Arnold Kegel, a Los Angeles gynecologist, was first to promote pelvic floor exercises and, hence, lent his name to them. He also invented the perineometer (peri-KNEE-ometer), a biofeedback device to measure the results of the exercises, which is still an important part of pelvic floor therapy today.

Even during Dr. Kegel's time, and for many years afterwards, very few health-care professionals saw the exercises as an alternative to surgery. For the most part, their use was largely confined to preparing women for natural childbirth, such as the Lamaze program, and, peripherally, for treating sexual dysfunction. Both applications of the exercises were on the right track. Unfortunately, mothers tended to stop the exercises after they gave birth. And, while mentioned in the literature, the sexual benefits of the Kegels have been explained away by some health-care professionals, perhaps blushingly, as an "oh by the way that's nice, but my dear it isn't what we're really here for now is it" side effect. But all that is changing. More and more health-care professionals in our fields have recognized the great potential benefits of these exercises.

The sexual benefits of doing the Kegels are real, as they're a critically important part of pelvic floor health. Pelvic floor therapy owes a debt of gratitude to Dr. Kegel for his early recognition and treatment of the problem. But we have taken it far beyond Kegels.

DON'T STOP WHEN YOU'RE AHEAD

Let's suppose that you choose pelvic floor therapy and you work at it conscientiously. You've found your pelvic floor and are beginning to "Unlock the Power of Your Secret Squeeze." You soon find that you're doing much better and you're enjoying *being* better – no more urgency, no more leaking. You have reached a critical point in your therapy.

Now let's suppose that you begin to let things slide. You return to your old ways. You stop the pelvic floor exercises, go back to drinking too much coffee, and maybe start smoking again. You really don't want to slip back to the bad old days of absorbent pads and so-so sex, but you're letting it happen anyway. After awhile, your symptoms reappear. Know why? You've skipped the last step: Commitment for Life.

This is for life.

The bladder urgency and urinary incontinence that you will learn to overcome had been a lifetime sentence of embarrassment and inconvenience. And don't forget the rewards in the bedroom. Please don't let the strength and control you've worked for slip away from you. Pelvic floor muscles are no different than other muscles that you exercise regularly. Abandon them and they will soon abandon you. Just like any other part of your body, your pelvic floor will continue to work well for you if you continue to treat it well. Keep an eye on your diet, forgo cigarettes, and exercise regularly. Moderation is the key. If you commit yourself to a healthier lifestyle, The Sisterhood Plan will set you free – without hard labor.

You won't get any benefits from the exercises unless you do them often and regularly. New mothers aren't the only ones who drop out of the program after everything has settled back into place; some of our incontinent patients also give up too soon. Despite the obvious benefits of the exercises, many women lose focus and stop after an initial period. At the first signs of improvement, they cease training, evidently unaware that the muscles will atrophy again and leave them back where they started. When you stop exercising, the decline begins immediately. It won't happen overnight, but most, if not all, of your gains will be lost. The bottom line: If you stop, you can expect your problem to return.

Other women just give up before they see results. Among the reasons they give us for dropping out is "it didn't work." In all probability, it didn't work for them because they weren't doing the exercises correctly. It's not uncommon for a patient to be pushing down on her pelvic floor muscles instead of contracting them. If somewhere along the way you've lost touch with your pelvic floor, it's time to see your health-care professional – or follow the instructions in this book to get back into it. We'll do everything we can to ensure that you're doing the exercises correctly and effectively.

If for whatever reason the therapy fails, it raises the question: Is there something about the exercises that discourage their continuation? We don't think so. We guarantee that you won't even break a sweat. The pelvic floor exercises take only a short amount of time about twice a day. You don't need a membership to a gym or any special equipment. You have all you need to get started right now. You can do them whenever you like and wherever you are. When you follow The Sisterhood Plan conscientiously, you will begin to experience improvement in a matter of weeks.

So, why would anyone stop the exercises just when they start seeing some improvement? Well, why does anybody give up exercising? They get bored with it, lose motivation, and let other things get in the way. What's usually missing is an individualized exercise program, based on what *you* can do, one that meets *your* individual needs and gets results for *you*. You will find such a program in The Sisterhood Plan – made for you – and it won't be burdensome or complicated.

What's more, you'll find the support you need on our Web site – *www.AccidentalSisterhood.com*. We'll be there to answer your questions and encourage action. You can also share your success story with other members of the Sisterhood who, like you, are finding their way along the path to pelvic floor health.

When you follow all of the steps of The Sisterhood Plan you'll begin to experience improvement of your problem in about four to six weeks. But, please, don't even consider stopping the exercises or forgetting all you learned about modifying your behavior or training your bladder. You must be committed to continue – especially the exercises.

It may take at least six months to *fully* correct a lifetime of being unaware of a fundamental part of your self, to turn bad bladder habits into good bladder habits, and rebuild the muscles of your pelvic floor. Considering the benefits, that's not a lot to ask of yourself for a lifetime solution. Once you begin to experience the improvement of your urgency and incontinence and, yes, your *sexual satisfaction*, you will want to – as you *must* – continue the training throughout all of your lifelong days. And that goes for every woman.

The message is clear: you have the power to improve the outcome of your treatment in every way. This is what we're going to ask you to do to be successful:

❀ Re-educate your bladder.

❀ Keep a fluid intake and voiding diary.

❀ Find the muscles of your pelvic floor.

❀ Create a Personal Progressive Exercise Plan.

❀ Follow your Personal Plan regularly.

❀ Give up the things that irritate your bladder.

❀ Remember to keep on doing what you've learned.

THE ACCIDENTAL SISTERHOOD PROGRESSIVE PLAN
— The Empowering Guide to Pelvic Floor Health —

{ Getting Organized }
*The Fluid Intake & Voiding Diary . . . The Baseline Strength
and Personal Progressive Exercise Log*

As you begin The Sisterhood Plan, one of the most important things we ask you to do is to chart your progress every day. Your success depends on how faithfully you keep and follow two very important records:

❀ Fluid Intake & Voiding Diary

❀ Baseline Strength and Personal Progressive Exercise Log

Please don't be alarmed. They don't require a great amount of record keeping. And they're indispensable to your success with the program.

The Voiding Diary and Exercise Log (see next page) are included as a companion piece to this book. It's a discreet journal for you to take with you and use every day as you work at The Sisterhood Plan. The journal also includes brief instructions and a list of bladder irritants, which includes the foods and beverages best avoided as you retrain your bladder. If you don't have a journal, you can get a copy at *www.AccidentalSisterhood.com*.

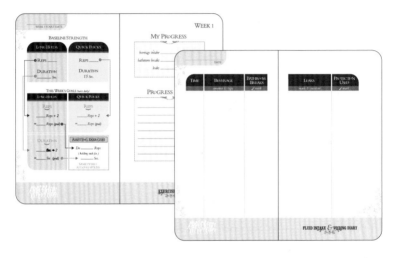

(Purse or pocket-sized, the Voiding Diary and Exercise Log are your personal and discreet records and reminders of your progress on The Sisterhood Plan.)

First, let's explain the Fluid Intake & Voiding Diary.

THE FLUID INTAKE & VOIDING DIARY

The Fluid Intake & Voiding Diary keeps track of how much you drink and how frequently you urinate and leak. It will reveal the extent of your problem and is an important first step in regaining bladder control. As you work on reducing your symptoms, the Diary helps you monitor your progress. Keeping a record of how frequently you urinate and how much you drink helps you understand how your body processes liquids. Best of all, you'll begin to notice significant strides in your progress, and nothing motivates better than seeing results.

Let's take another look at the Voiding Diary and review the instructions:

Instructions for the Fluid Intake & Voiding Diary:

(1) Record the date: Each day should begin at midnight. Remember to record both day and nighttime activity.

(2) Record what you drink: In the "Beverages" column, identify what you drank and when. Record how much you drank.

(3) Record your bathroom visits: In the "Bathroom Breaks" column, place a check (✓) next to each time you went to the bathroom. Use an asterisk (★) to note times when you were awakened from sleep to go to the bathroom.

(4) Record your leaks: Place a check (✓) next to the times you noticed leakage and describe them, using words like "small" or "large," and what you were doing when they happened, such as lifting, coughing, or having a sudden urge.

(5) Record your protection: Write down the number of pads you used during the day, not each time you changed it during the day. Also note the degree of saturation.

(See the Voiding Diary illustration on the next page; the numbers above each column correspond with the numbered instructions.)

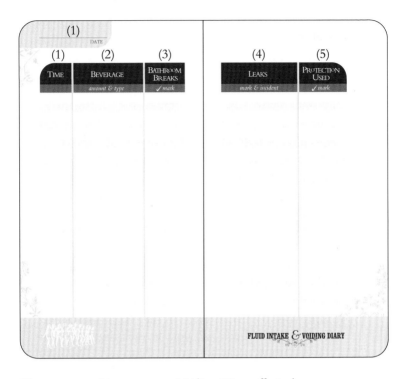

			(1) _____ DATE		
(1)	(2)	(3)		(4)	(5)
TIME	BEVERAGE	BATHROOM BREAKS		LEAKS	PROTECTION USED
	amount & type	*✓ mark*		*mark & incident*	*✓ mark*

FLUID INTAKE *&* VOIDING DIARY

How to use and interpret your Voiding Diary effectively:

✤ When you look over your Diary, take note of how often you're urinating. Your goal is to urinate between five and eight times a day, including zero to only once during the night.

✤ You want to drink from six to eight eight-ounce glasses of a non-irritating fluid throughout the day. You *don't* want to drink a lot of fluid each time you drink.

✤ By monitoring when you drink and how much you drink, you may discover that you drink too much and/or too often. That may be why you leak an hour later or have to get up three times during the night.

✤ You may also find that you're not drinking enough fluid. The Voiding Diary will help you adjust your fluid intake up or down, which may go a long way toward helping you control the urges.

❀ By monitoring how much you leak and what you might be doing when it happens, you may be able to avoid certain activities until you get stronger. Or you might do a pelvic floor contraction during these activities to reduce the leaks. You can find techniques to help you control urges in the section **Bladder Training**.

❀ You'll find that you're having fewer leaks over the weeks to come, and your Voiding Diary will serve as a reminder of how "it used to be."

Here's an example of an actual Fluid Intake & Voiding Diary recorded by a patient:

4/25/07
DATE

Time	Beverage amount & type	Bathroom Breaks ✓ mark	Leaks mark & incident	Protection Used ✓ mark
2am		✓		✓
4:30am		✓		new pad (dry)
7am	2oz water			
8am	8oz coffee			
8:30am		✓		
10am	4oz coffee	✓	✓ coughed -sm. leak	
11:30am		✓		
12pm	12oz diet soda			
3:30pm	12oz bottled water	✓	✓ sudden urge - lg. leak	✓ change pad -wet
5pm		✓		
6pm	8oz milk	✓		
7pm				
8pm	3oz water	✓		
9:30pm			✓ while getting up - med.	✓ change pad
11pm		✓		
		✓		✓ new pad for night

FLUID INTAKE & VOIDING DIARY

Other examples can be found online at *www.AccidentalSisterhood.com*. Again, keeping the Voiding Diary faithfully will prove to be very beneficial to your pelvic floor therapy.

THE BASELINE STRENGTH AND PERSONAL PROGRESSIVE EXCERCISE LOG

The Baseline Strength and Personal Progressive Exercise Log is designed to show you:

❋ How to start your Personal Progressive Exercise Plan.

❋ How to set new strength goals for each week.

❋ How well you've progressed.

The Exercise Log (shown on the right) is a week-to-week snapshot of your progress in strengthening your pelvic floor muscles.

The Exercise Log will also help you evaluate your progress on bladder control as you follow your exercise regimen. But before we discuss how to use the Exercise Log, there are a number of important things you need to know first. They're covered in the next section.

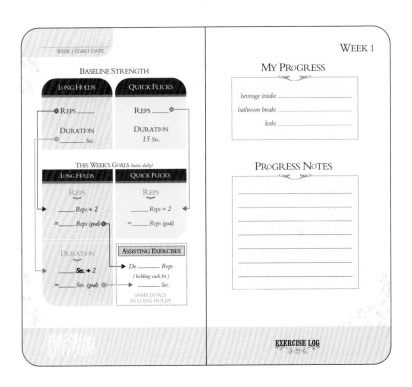

WEEK 1 START DATE

BASELINE STRENGTH

LONG HOLDS **QUICK FLICKS**

REPS _____ REPS _____

DURATION _____ Sec. DURATION 15 Sec.

THIS WEEK'S GOALS *(twice daily)*

LONG HOLDS **QUICK FLICKS**

REPS REPS

_____ Reps + 2 _____ Reps + 2

= _____ Reps (goal) = _____ Reps (goal)

DURATION **ASSISTING EXERCISES**

_____ Sec. + 2 Do _____ Reps

= _____ Sec. (goal) *(holding each for)*

_____ Sec.

SAME GOALS
AS LONG HOLDS

WEEK 1

MY PROGRESS

beverage intake _____
bathroom breaks _____
leaks _____

PROGRESS NOTES

_____
_____
_____
_____
_____
_____
_____

EXERCISE LOG

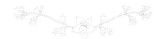

THE ACCIDENTAL SISTERHOOD PROGRESSIVE PLAN
— *The Empowering Guide to Pelvic Floor Health* —

{ Progressive Pelvic Floor Exercises }

*Find – and Feel – Your Pelvic Floor . . . The Long Hold and The Quick
Flicks . . . Assisting Exercises . . . Setting Up Your Personal Progressive
Exercise Log . . . The Fifty-Percent Strength Progression*

FIND – AND FEEL – YOUR PELVIC FLOOR

As we've described, the pelvic floor is a hammock of muscles
that supports your pelvic organs: the bladder, uterus, vagina, and
rectum. The most common types of urinary incontinence are
directly linked to a woman's weak pelvic floor muscles.

The good news is that, barring any severe neurological
problem, the pelvic floor muscles can usually be strengthened to
end incontinence.

First, find the pelvic floor muscles. Since you can't see these muscles,
you need to learn how to feel them in order to exercise them.

Here are some ways to help you recognize where and when these muscles are working:

* The next time you're on the toilet, stop the stream of urine. You may not be able to stop the stream completely, but you will feel the area where you need to concentrate your efforts. (Please Note: Only use this as a test to find the pelvic floor muscles. Doing it too often can cause bladder problems.)

* Feel the muscles firsthand. Prop yourself up in bed, leaning slightly back. Slowly and gently insert two moistened fingers into your vagina. Contract or pull up your muscles, as if you're trying to pull your fingers inside you. You should be able to feel some movement around your fingers. If it doesn't work, try this:

~ Imagine what it would feel like if you had to pass gas in a crowded elevator and you're trying not to make a sound – only don't squeeze your buttock cheeks together. Just squeeze your pelvic floor muscles.

* (If you have symptoms of stress urinary incontinence, this exercise might cause you to leak, so be prepared.) With your fingers inside you, cough or bear down as if you're having a bowel movement. You should feel a downward movement, exactly opposite from doing a pelvic floor contraction. Now: quickly pull up and inward. You may feel some pressure around the tips of your fingers.

You'll know if you're doing the exercises correctly if you feel a lifting and tightening of the muscles around the vagina, from the pubic bone to the small of your back. Don't tighten the large buttock muscles (*gluteus muscles*) or your abdominal muscles; instead, concentrate on the area around your vagina.

Use the following techniques to confirm that you're contracting the correct muscles:

* Hold a mirror between your legs to see the perineum move

upwards when you contract your muscles. Or place the tips of your fingers in this area and feel the muscles contract inward.

❁ Try the squeeze with your partner. Squeeze your pelvic floor muscles. Ask your partner if he feels any pressure with his fingers or penis inside you. Discuss how strong your squeeze is at first, then ask for additional feedback as time passes, when it's likely that he'll feel a stronger response. This can be a great motivator.

❁ Try the squeeze *without* a partner. Lubricate a tampon and insert it. Try to tighten around it and feel the resistance as you attempt to pull it out.

If after trying all of these ways to feel your pelvic floor muscles you're still unsuccessful, you should seek the help of a physical therapist, specifically one who specializes in pelvic floor training. A therapist can help you by using biofeedback and very-low-power-level electrical stimulation. For more about these and other measures to help you improve your progress, turn to **Devices . . . and Desire**.

THE LONG HOLD AND THE QUICK FLICKS

Two types of contractions strengthen the muscles of the pelvic floor, the Long Hold, an endurance contraction, and the Quick Flicks, rapid-response contractions. There are two kinds of exercise contractions because pelvic floor muscles are made up of two types of muscle fibers, slow twitch and fast twitch.

The Long Hold strengthens the slow-twitch muscle fibers, which provide the constant, resting tone that supports the weight and pressure of the pelvic organs. Seventy percent of your pelvic floor muscles are slow-twitch fibers.

The Quick Flicks strengthen the fast-twitch muscle fibers, which account for the remaining 30 percent of the muscle fibers. These muscle fibers are needed to respond quickly when you cough or sneeze or lift a heavy object – any action that exerts an intra-abdominal pressure on your bladder. These contractions act to provide reflex inhibition of bladder contraction.

These muscles – the slow-twitch and the fast-twitch – work in unison at all times to give the pelvic floor a stable base to help keep the urethra from leaking and to be able to respond quickly and firmly to resist a sudden pressure exerted on the bladder.

It's important that you learn how to do each of these important exercises correctly. You can do Long Holds and Quick Flicks lying down, sitting up, or standing. We recommend that beginners start lying down and work up to the standing position, which is the most challenging.

The first thing we're going to ask you to do is to find your baseline strengths for each exercise. This is important, as you will see later on.

The Long Hold

Find your baseline strength by lying down and counting the seconds you can hold a strong contraction. Try for at least two seconds – a sneeze or a cough can last that long. Many women can hold a contraction for only a second or two, while others may be able to hold one for 10 seconds or longer.

If you can hold a strong squeeze, please don't imagine that

these exercises aren't for you. Many women have what initially seems to be a strong pelvic floor, but in fact it doesn't function properly to control urination and other bladder-control issues. As strong as your pelvic floor may seem to be, it will still benefit from and respond to continual exercise.

Don't kid yourself. If you're holding for as long as 30 seconds, the strength of your squeeze has probably fallen off. Either you aren't squeezing as hard as you can, or you're relaxing from a strong initial squeeze into a light squeeze. In any case, don't over-estimate your hold time. This isn't a competition. And remember not to use muscles that can be seen to move, like your buttocks or abdomen. You want to do a good, solid squeeze; don't hold your breath or use any other muscles.

How many Long Holds can you do? Repeat the squeeze and hold, relax, rest for five seconds, and repeat as many times as you can until your muscles feel too weak to continue. Do not use your abdominal muscles to help. Remember to keep breathing during the exercise. *This is your Baseline Strength.*

Don't be discouraged if you can't repeat the contraction more than a few times. The muscles are weak, but they'll strengthen quickly as you do the exercises. You'll find that you'll also be able to reach and hold stronger contractions over a longer period of time. These exercises will help train pelvic floor muscles to function better from wherever on the strength scale you are when you start exercising.

And by the way, the resting time between contractions is important. Weak muscles need a little more time to recover. Rest may prevent the discomfort that some women report as they begin the exercises. Exercise can make any muscle sore, so it's important to start out gradually and avoid overusing the muscles as you strengthen them.

{ Hold/Rest Ratio Varies }

As your pelvic floor muscles gain strength and you can do more repetitions, the resting period will vary. Typically, at the start, we rest our muscles between contractions for five seconds. But as your strength increases, the contraction/rest ratio becomes more equal, until when we can hold for 10 seconds, we rest for 10 seconds, and so on.

The Quick Flicks

The Quick Flicks are a series of strong, quick contractions in rapid succession. These great exercises build the strength of the pelvic floor muscles that are needed to quickly shut off the flow of urine. You must strengthen these fast-twitch muscle fibers because they're necessary to keep you dry when you laugh, sneeze, or cough.

Let's try some Quick Flicks. First, find your baseline strength while lying down and doing Quick Flicks in rapid succession with no rest between them. You're doing them correctly if you squeeze hard, then just as quickly relax all the way. Then quickly, squeeze hard again, relax all the way, and so on. Don't flutter the muscles. That's not doing Quick Flicks. See how many Quick Flicks you can feel before the muscles tire, or you reach 15 seconds. *That's your current limit, or Baseline Strength.*

Now you know where your pelvic muscles stand. You know how many Long Holds you can do and how long you can hold them. And you know how many Quick Flicks you can do in rapid succession. Now you know your Baseline Strengths. More about this later.

Now choose two of the Assisting Pelvic Floor Muscle Exercises listed and do the same number of each of them as you do for the Long Hold contraction.

Assisting Exercises

Each of the following exercises is designed to assist your pelvic floor muscles in recruiting additional muscle fibers. By that we mean reaching out and incorporating new reserves of strength to help the muscles perform more efficiently, especially their reflexes, which are called upon when you cough or sneeze.

Just doing the Long Holds and Quick Flicks will build your strength, but adding additional exercises will help you gain greater strength, endurance, and coordination.

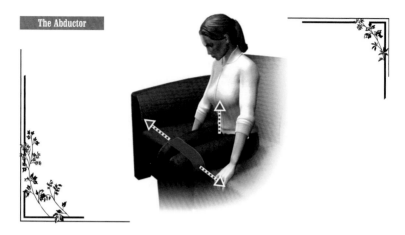

The Abductor *(See illustration)*

What it does: The Abductor exercise strengthens the muscles found just above the pelvic floor on both of the inner sides of the pelvis, in addition to increasing the strength of the pelvic floor muscles.

Additional benefits: This exercise helps stabilize the lower back and can reduce lower back pain, while toning hips and thighs.

Position options: You can do this exercise either lying down with knees bent or sitting with good posture (as shown).

Two ways to do it: One: Tie the two ends of an elastic resistive exercise band around your thighs, keeping the band near your knees. The tighter the loop around your legs, the more resistance you'll work against. Now pull your legs apart while doing a Long Hold, keeping your feet together and feeling the resistance offered by the band. Don't let your ankles come apart very far, and don't forget to breathe.

Two: If you don't have a band, lie down on your back or sit in a chair with proper posture. Bend your knees, keeping your ankles together and your feet flat on the bed or floor. Place your hands on the outside of your knees and, while doing a Long Hold, press your knees together as you push them outward.

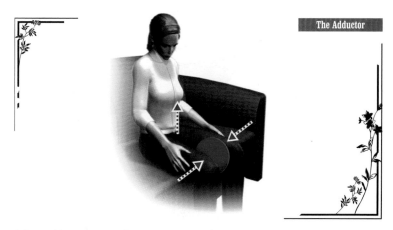

The Adductor

The Adductor *(See illustration)*

What it does: The Adductor strengthens the muscles on the inside of the thighs.

Additional benefits: This exercise helps stabilize the lower back and can reduce lower back pain while toning hips and thighs.

Position options: You can do this exercise either lying down with knees bent or sitting with good posture (as shown).

How to do it: Bend your knees, keeping your ankles six to eight inches apart, and place a pillow or your hands together between your knees. Now, without using your hands, press your knees together while doing a Long Hold. A rolled-up towel or a small ball between your knees can also offer resistance to the pressure from your knees.

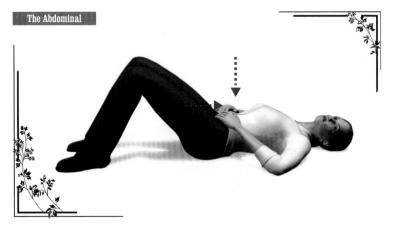

The Abdominal *(See illustration)*

What it does: The Abdominal strengthens the abdominal muscles that span your entire lower torso, specifically the lower abs, and helps strengthen pelvic stability.

Additional benefits: This exercise may improve posture and tone your lower abdomen.

How to do it: You can do this exercise lying down (as shown) or sitting with proper posture. Lie with your legs bent, or sit with your legs bent and your back straight. Place your hands on your lower abdomen below your belly button and your hipbones so you can feel the muscle working. Take in a deep breath, and as you let it out, pull your lower abdomen in toward your spine as if you're pulling on a pair of jeans one size too small. Keep your back straight and concentrate on the movement you feel in the lower part of your abdomen. At the same time, do a Long Hold. Don't push down. Hold the contraction of the abdominal muscle and your pelvic floor contraction until you completely exhale. If you begin doing this exercise while lying down, progress to sitting as the exercise becomes easier.

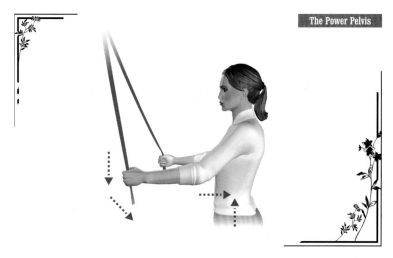

The Power Pelvis

The Power Pelvis *(See illustration)*

What it does: The Power Pelvis is great for those who have mastered the Long Hold, the Quick Flicks, the abdominal exercises, and are ready for something new. This exercise helps stabilize the lower back, abdominals, and pelvic region.

Additional benefits: The Power Pelvis improves posture, enhances mind/body awareness, and engages more muscle fibers in the pelvic floor for improved strength.

How to do it: Secure the resistive elastic band above you from the top of a door, with the two ends hanging down. (You should tie a knot in the middle of the band and place it over the top of the door, closing the door to secure it. But be careful. If it isn't placed securely, the band may snap down and hit you in the face.) To start, face the door, reach up and grasp each end of the band. Stand up tall, tuck your buttocks underneath you (the pelvic tilt), and pull your abdomen in, as you'd do while pulling on a pair of tight jeans. Now, do a pelvic floor muscle contraction and keep your arms straight while you slowly lower them to your side, pulling against the resistive band. Hold this position for five to 10 seconds, then slowly return to the starting position.

Okay. You've mastered the Long Hold and the Quick Flicks. You've tried out the Assisting Exercises and there are a couple of them that you like. You're now ready to begin your pelvic floor muscle-strengthening program. But first, let's set up your Baseline Strength and Personal Progressive Exercise Log.

Baseline Strength and Personal Progressive Exercise Log

You learned earlier that the Long Hold and the Quick Flicks exercise two types of voluntary muscle fiber found in all pelvic floor muscles. One type is essential to maintaining the tone of the pelvic floor muscles, which is exercised by the Long Hold. The other type allows the muscles to respond quickly to shut off the plumbing when you cough or sneeze, which is exercised by the Quick Flicks.

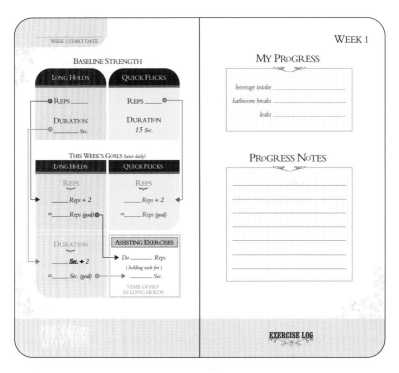

As you can see on your Exercise Log, we ask you to add two Assisting Exercises each week. You get to choose the ones you want to do. Refer back to **Assisting Exercises** to help you make your choices.

How to Use Your Exercise Log
Part One: Establish your Baseline Strengths.

If you've already tested yourself on the Long Hold and the Quick Flicks, you know what your Baseline Strengths are. If not, you can do so now. You are asked to perform these two strength-testing exercises to establish your Baseline Strengths at the start of your progressive exercise therapy and, then again, each week thereafter:

- Start with Long Holds – contract and hold your pelvic floor muscles for as long as you can hold a good squeeze without slipping. *This is how you measure your Long Hold Baseline Strength.*

- Record how long you held your Long Hold squeeze and how many times you can repeat that exact same squeeze, until you can't do another. Be sure to rest five seconds between squeezes. This is your Baseline Strength.

- Next, do the Quick Flicks – contract your pelvic floor muscles as hard as you can, relax, and squeeze again in rapid succession *to measure your Quick Flicks Baseline Strength.*

- Record how many Quick Flicks you can do in 15 seconds to find your Baseline Strength.

Part Two: Set your goals.

Write your plan goals, based on 50 percent, or half, of your Baseline Strengths, at the beginning of the first week. For more details on how to calculate your Baseline Strength from week to week, see **The Fifty-Percent Strength Progression** section.

Next, at the beginning of each week, referring to your Fluid Intake & Voiding Diary, write down the previous week's average daily:

- Beverage Intake
- Bathroom Breaks
- Leaks

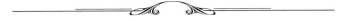

{ First Thing First }
We recommend that you maintain a Voiding Diary for
three to seven days before you start The Sisterhood Plan.

Obviously, the reason we want you to keep such a record is to show you that, as you're getting stronger each week, you're also making progress toward staying dry. Study the sample of the Exercise Log in this section or visit our Web site for more samples. The increasing strength of your pelvic floor will also begin to show up as a *decreasing* average number of urinations and leaks, and these are the results that tell you The Sisterhood Plan is working for you.
Do all of your exercises – the Long Hold, the Quick Flicks, and do any two Assisting Exercises – once or twice a day. And at the end of Week One, start ramping it up, as we explain in the next section.

(Sample Logs are shown on next page spread, progressively showing the baseline Long Holds and Quick Flicks results and the average daily values taken from previous weeks' Fluid Intake & Voiding Diary.)

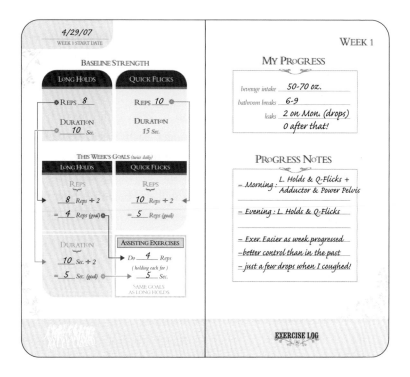

4/29/07
WEEK 1 START DATE

BASELINE STRENGTH

LONG HOLDS | **QUICK FLICKS**

REPS *8* | REPS *10*

DURATION
10 Sec. | DURATION
15 Sec.

THIS WEEK'S GOALS *(twice daily)*

LONG HOLDS | **QUICK FLICKS**

REPS | REPS

8 Reps ÷ 2 | *10* Reps ÷ 2

= *4* Reps (goal) | = *5* Reps (goal)

DURATION | **ASSISTING EXERCISES**

10 Sec. ÷ 2 | Do *4* Reps
(holding each for)
= *5* Sec. (goal) | *5* Sec.

| SAME GOALS
AS LONG HOLDS

MY PROGRESS

beverage intake *50-70 oz.*
bathroom breaks *6-9*
leaks *2 on Mon. (drops)*
0 after that!

PROGRESS NOTES

– *Morning :* *L. Holds & Q-Flicks +*
Adductor & Power Pelvis

– *Evening : L. Holds & Q-Flicks*

– *Exer. Easier as week progressed*
– *better control than in the past*
– *just a few drops when I coughed!*

EXERCISE LOG

THE FIFTY-PERCENT STRENGTH PROGRESSION

Because this is a *progressive* exercise plan, you will build up your strength gradually, based on your current level of strength. To do that, start exercising at 50 percent of your initial Baseline Strength for both the Long Hold and the Quick Flicks. *The reasoning behind this is simple: If you try to do your utmost at the beginning of an exercise program, it can make your pelvic muscles sore and delay your progress.*

{ Progressive Pelvic Floor Exercises }

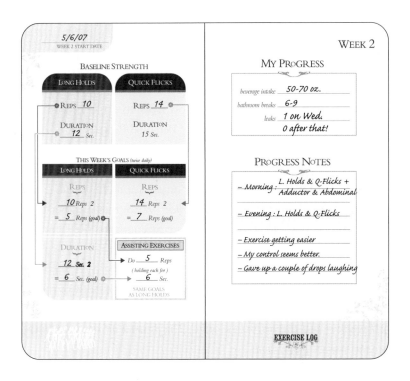

BASELINE STRENGTH

LONG HOLDS	QUICK FLICKS
✸ REPS _10_	REPS _14_ ✸
DURATION	DURATION
✸ _12_ Sec.	15 Sec.

THIS WEEK'S GOALS *(twice daily)*

LONG HOLDS	QUICK FLICKS
REPS	REPS
_10_ Reps 2	_14_ Reps 2
= _5_ Reps (goal) ✸	= _7_ Reps (goal)

DURATION	ASSISTING EXERCISES
_12_ Sec. 2	▶ Do _5_ Reps
= _6_ Sec. (goal) ✸	*(holding each for)* ▶ _6_ Sec.
	SAME GOALS AS LONG HOLDS

MY PROGRESS

beverage intake	50-70 oz.
bathroom breaks	6-9
leaks	1 on Wed.
	0 after that!

PROGRESS NOTES

– *Morning* : L. Holds & Q-Flicks + Adductor & Abdominal

– *Evening* : L. Holds & Q-Flicks

– *Exercise getting easier*

– *My control seems better.*

– *Gave up a couple of drops laughing*

EXERCISE LOG

The Importance of Baseline Strength

Let's suppose that you were to go see a personal trainer at the gym. She would probably start your first consultation by measuring your strength. You'd be asked to lift as much weight as you can and for as many reps as you can before your muscles give up. And while you may be thinking, "Wow, this is a killer workout," the purpose of this initial test is to create fitness goals based on a *percentage of your maximum* performance. At your next visit, the weight you'll lift will be lighter so that you can safely and effectively build your muscle strength without overdoing it. You'll take this same approach with your pelvic floor exercise.

Remember: To find your Baseline Strength, you'll hold a Long Hold for as long as possible before your muscles give out. You'll rest five seconds, then do another Long Hold and repeat the exercise until your muscles feel too weak to do any more. Record the *hold time* and *reps* in your Personal Progressive Exercise Log. *That's your Baseline Strength for the Long Hold.*

For the Quick Flicks, *do as many as you can in 15 seconds—and no pauses allowed between each Quick Flick.* Write that number in your Exercise Log. That's your Baseline Strength for the Quick Flicks.

Now, this is where the math comes in. Divide both of these Baseline Strength numbers in half. These are your goals for the *first* week – and the *first* week only. *This is what we mean by "fifty-percent strength progression."*

Confused? Use the following examples for reference:

Long Holds

- ❀ Your Baseline Strength for a Long Hold was four seconds.

- ❀ You could do *six four-second* Long Holds, resting five seconds between each, before your muscles felt too weak to go on and you stopped.

- ❀ Your goal for the *first* week: *Three two-second* Long Holds.

Quick Flicks

* ❋ You can do 10 Quick Flicks in 15 seconds at the beginning of Week One. This is your Baseline Strength.

* ❋ Your goal for the *first* week: *Five* Quick Flicks in 15 seconds.

Your level of strength should change each week, and that is why *you will test and record your new Baseline Strengths each week.* Test your Baseline Strengths in both exercises and set new goals at the beginning of every week. You should feel a gradual increase in your times and reps.

Go to the next sample of the Exercise Log (next page). Note that in Week Two, the goals are 50 percent of your *new* Baseline Strengths for the Long Hold and the Quick Flicks.

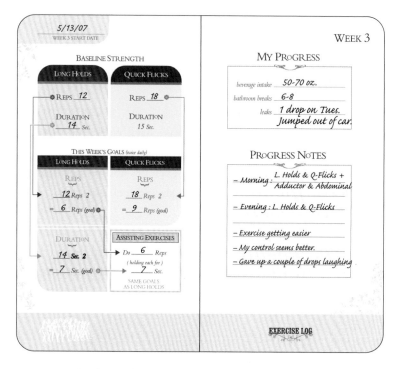

5/13/07
WEEK 3 START DATE

BASELINE STRENGTH

LONG HOLDS | QUICK FLICKS

REPS _12_

REPS _18_

DURATION
_14_ Sec.

DURATION
15 Sec.

THIS WEEK'S GOALS *(twice daily)*

LONG HOLDS | QUICK FLICKS

REPS
_12_ Reps 2
= _6_ Reps *(goal)*

REPS
_18_ Reps 2
= _9_ Reps *(goal)*

DURATION
_14_ Sec. 2
= _7_ Sec. *(goal)*

ASSISTING EXERCISES
Do _6_ Reps
(holding each for)
_7_ Sec.
SAME GOALS
AS LONG HOLDS

MY PROGRESS

beverage intake _50-70 oz._
bathroom breaks _6-8_
leaks _1 drop on Tues._
Jumped out of car.

PROGRESS NOTES

– Morning : *L. Holds & Q-Flicks +*
Adductor & Abdominal

– Evening : *L. Holds & Q-Flicks*

– *Exercise getting easier*
– *My control seems better.*
– *Gave up a couple of drops laughing*

EXERCISE LOG

In Week Three, the goals are ramped up again as your Baseline Strengths increase. Again, they're 50 percent of your new and increasing Baseline Strengths. And so on – in Week Four, Five, Six, Seven, and so forth. Get the idea? The word is gradual. You're working on the progressive strengthening of your pelvic floor muscles.

Okay, so you're doing the exercises at least twice a day. Right? And you're continuing to build on each week's goal (50 percent at a time) until you've surpassed your original Baseline Strengths. From then on, keep raising your Baseline Strengths to the level that maintains your positive results.

{ Progressive Pelvic Floor Exercises }

And don't forget to add two Assisting Exercises to your workout. Do any two. Alternate them as you wish. But do them.

At this point, you've learned to use two essential tools to build and retain pelvic floor strength – The Fluid Intake & Voiding Diary and The Personal Progressive Exercise Log. The information in the following sections – Bladder Training and Behavior Modification – will enable you to make even more progress on your road to improved pelvic floor health and fitness.

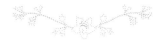

THE ACCIDENTAL SISTERHOOD PROGRESSIVE PLAN
— *The Empowering Guide to Pelvic Floor Health* —

{ Bladder Training }

A Healthy Bladder is a Wondrous Thing . . .
Taking Back Control . . . Put Your Bladder on a Schedule . . .
Believe in Yourself. Believe That You Can Do It. . . . The Knack

A HEALTHY BLADDER IS A WONDROUS THING

Maybe you remember when your bladder was healthy. You didn't have to think about it all the time, and it worked as easily as breathing. When it was full, you knew it was full, no problem. As a kid, you could put off going until the game was over. Holding on, you could run home and get into the bathroom in plenty of time without a drop escaping. As you matured, you never gave your bladder a second thought, unless you had to go. Even then, you could easily hold on until a bathroom was convenient. But then, as the years went by, your bladder started to become more insistent. The signals were coming more often and they were stronger. They gave you no peace. And now there's the leaking.

You don't want to believe that what's happening to you is normal. Well, you're right; it isn't. Here's how a normal bladder behaves:

- ❀ Urges are not commands. An urge to urinate is a signal from your bladder as it stretches to fill with urine. Urges can be felt even if the bladder is not full.

- ❀ Typically, during a normal 24-hour day, you should urinate every two to five hours, with an average of five to eight trips to the bathroom.

- ❀ Your bladder stores urine by relaxing and allowing the urine to collect and expels urine by contracting fully.

- ❀ The average bladder holds about two cups (16 ounces) of urine before it needs to be emptied. Your stream should last at least 10 to 15 seconds.

- ❀ Urine should flow easily without discomfort in a good, steady stream until the bladder is empty. No pushing or straining is necessary to empty the bladder.

When you feel the urge to urinate, you're getting a signal that passes between your bladder and your brain. With some training, you'll be able to suppress the urge. You don't have to be a passive participant in this process; you can use your brain to contract your pelvic floor muscles to make your bladder behave the way it's supposed to behave.

Let's start the bladder retraining process by describing good bladder habits:

- ❀ You take your time when emptying your bladder. You don't strain or push to empty your bladder. Sometimes you lean forward as you go; it helps to make sure your bladder is completely empty each time you urinate. You take your time and don't rush.

- ❀ You don't go to the bathroom before you leave the house or whenever you pass the ladies' room while out shopping "just in case." You almost never go just to keep your bladder empty.

As for bad bladder habits, just-in-case urinating is one of the main culprits in causing urinary frequency. The bladder has learned to signal the brain that it needs to urinate before it's full, ultimately leading to overactive bladder-dry. Your bladder begins to rule your brain and, ultimately, your life. It will signal the need to urinate and begin contractions to urinate with smaller and smaller amounts of urine. Although your bladder's capacity to hold urine remains the same, it starts acting as if it's full, even when it isn't. And pretty soon you aren't getting to a bathroom in time.

Generally speaking, it isn't necessary to urinate when you feel the first urge. But there's a flip side to this coin: consistently ignoring the urge to go for long periods can be equally damaging. Urinating too infrequently may be convenient, but it isn't healthy for your bladder. And it may lead to symptoms of overflow incontinence.

And don't forget. Avoiding bladder irritants (See **Behavior Modification**) and drinking plenty of fluids are also important to the health of your bladder.

TAKING BACK CONTROL

The object of bladder training is to restore good bladder habits. The process requires a coordinated effort involving Behavior Modification, Pelvic Floor Exercises, and the Bladder Training techniques described in this section. As you learn these techniques and begin to apply them, you will regain voluntary control of your bladder and decrease inappropriate urge sensations and bladder contractions.

Learn to Control the Urge.

The following techniques will help you control urgency and will also help prevent leaking when you have a sudden or strong urge to urinate:

Stop right where you are.

- ❀ Stand very still and don't move.

- ❀ Focus on maintaining or regaining control of your urine and bladder.

- ❀ Sit if necessary. Sometimes this helps.

- ❀ Try crossing your legs or holding yourself between your legs to apply pressure to the perineum. (This technique may be helpful in the beginning but is not recommended for long-term urge suppression. And, of course, it usually isn't appropriate in most social situations.)

Relax.

- ❀ Try to make the urge go away by thinking of something other than going to the bathroom. That's a tough one, especially when you really have to go and go bad. Take your mind elsewhere.

- ❀ Take several deep breaths in through your nose and let them out through your mouth.

- ❀ Calm yourself. Since urges come in waves, they'll often decrease in intensity or go away if you relax.

Contract and squeeze.

- ❀ Tighten your pelvic floor muscles and hold for five seconds. (If you can't hold for five seconds, do multiple Quick Flicks.)

- ❀ Squeeze three or four more times to keep from leaking.

Walk.

- ❀ As the urge begins to fade, walk – don't run – to the bathroom.

- ❀ As you gain control, don't be too quick to think you're home free. If you're in a public place, you may have to wait a few minutes before you gain access to a stall.

- ❀ If the urge returns on your way to the bathroom, stop and repeat these techniques.

Even with practice, you may find that you're not always able to suppress an urge without leaking. Don't be discouraged. Your bladder has learned its very inconvenient behavior over many years, often a lifetime. Patience is needed as you retrain your bladder to function normally. It's also a good idea to start practicing these retraining techniques at home where you have access to a change of clothes or pads, just in case.

{ *What's Normal, Anyway?* }

It may be normal to urinate one hour or less after you drink a large amount of fluid. However, your total bathroom visits should still be five to eight times a day unless you're drinking more than 68 ounces of fluid – that's more than eight, eight-ounce glasses.

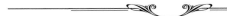

Put Your Bladder on a Schedule

Oftentimes, just being aware of your bladder – keeping a Voiding Diary, knowing how often you should be going to the bathroom (not just-in-case urinating), and learning to control your urges – is enough to decrease your voiding to five to eight times a day, a normal number. When it isn't, there are two timed-voiding schedules to try.

Below are two approaches to timed voiding – ways in which you can put your bladder on *your* schedule. The first one will help you increase the interval between urges. The second one will help you actively exert control over your bladder.

Try one approach first. Then move on to the second approach as you are able to reduce the number of urges.

Timed-Voiding Schedule – One

Goal: Your objective is to increase the time between bathroom breaks and train your bladder to hold more urine before it signals an urge to urinate.

Use your Fluid Intake & Voiding Diary to record how often you use the bathroom. If you notice that you frequently urinate in the morning when you get up and then again 30 minutes later, you would choose 30 minutes as your prescribed interval to wait between urinations. You should not allow yourself to go to the bathroom in less than 30 minutes. As you improve, you increase this time to 45 minutes and upward until you can hold your urine for two hours. You should increase your time intervals once each week.

You can also attempt this approach in this way: When you get the urge, stop, relax, contract, and wait five minutes. Soon, you'll be confident and comfortable to add five minutes to your time. Continue adding another five minutes until you're up to your two-hour goal.

Timed-Voiding Schedule – Two

Goal: Your objective is to go to the bathroom at a prescribed interval of time (for example, every hour) whether you have to go or not. This helps you exert voluntary control over your bladder and, ultimately, re-wire the neurological pathway from your brain to your bladder to regain control.

Start by choosing your bathroom schedule. For most women, it's usually around once every hour. But if you're among the many women who urinate more than 20 times a day, you'll need to start this exercise using 30-minute intervals. As you improve, you increase this time to 45 minutes and upward until you can hold your urine for two hours.

Here is an example of how Timed-Voiding Schedule – Two should work:

Week One

- ❀ Urinate when you first get out of bed in the morning. This is your initial start time. If you have a strong urge before you get out of bed, contract and squeeze the muscle that holds back your urine. Hold the squeeze for five seconds. Then walk to the bathroom.
- ❀ Empty your bladder as completely as you can and record the date and time that you urinated. Place a check (✓) in the Bathroom Breaks column.

❀ Set your kitchen timer for one hour or check your watch for the time an hour from now. When the hour is up, go to the bathroom even if you don't think you have to go. Place a check (✓) in the Bathroom Breaks column.

❀ Repeat this step again every hour throughout the day until you go to bed. No matter where you are. Remember to record the time each time you place a check in the Bathroom Breaks column.

❀ Record any Bathroom Breaks you may have had at night after you go to bed for future reference, but you don't need to urinate every hour. You should see your nighttime visits to the bathroom decrease.

Increase your time between Bathroom Breaks to the following intervals for the remainder of the timed-voiding plan:

Week Two: An hour and a half.

Week Three: One hour and 45 minutes.

Week Four: Two hours.

Week Five: Two and half hours.

Week Six: Three hours.

Tips for Success with Timed-Voiding Schedule – Two

❀ If you have a strong urge before you get out of bed, contract and squeeze the muscle that holds back your urine. Hold the squeeze for five seconds. Then walk to the bathroom.

❀ Practice urge control techniques at the beginning of every new week when you increase your time intervals.

❀ If you still have trouble increasing your time, don't get discouraged. Simply stay at the existing time for another week until you feel you're ready to advance.

{ Bladder Training }

❀ After a week or two, if you're finding it easy to postpone the scheduled urinations and your daily total has decreased to five to eight times, you've done it. Congratulations. If not, continue on the Week Three to Six schedule.

❀ Maintain your Voiding Diary faithfully.

❀ Don't forget to record your averages in the Baseline Strength and Personal Progressive Exercise Log to note your progress as you exercise.

BELIEVE IN YOURSELF.
BELIEVE THAT YOU CAN DO IT.

❀ Give The Sisterhood Plan's Bladder Training program a full six weeks or more.

❀ Stick to it. Be patient if you're not progressing as well as you think you should. There will be setbacks, and that's normal, especially when you're tired, tense, or expecting your period. Cold, rainy days can be difficult for you, too.

❀ Drink plenty of fluids, up to eight glasses of water or other non-irritating beverages every day. This is especially important in gaining control.

❀ Take care of your bowel habits. Constipation can put extra pressure on your bladder. Add fiber to your diet. You need about 30 grams of dietary fiber every day. (See **Healthy Bowel Function** and **Fiber Facts** in the **Appendix**.)

❀ Avoid the bladder irritants we list in the **Behavior Modification** section.

❀ Practice the urge control techniques as often as necessary.

❀ And most important, don't reinforce old bladder habits by going to the bathroom "just in case." Except while you're re-training your bladder to go on your command, if you have no need to go, then don't. If you feel that your bladder is slightly or moderately full and you don't expect a bathroom to be within your reach for at least two hours, then go ahead and urinate. Delaying a strong urge to urinate isn't good, either.

Bladder Training is essential to The Sisterhood Plan. If done conscientiously and in conjunction with Behavior Modification (in the next section) and the Progressive Pelvic Floor Exercises, it will accelerate your therapy. These three initiatives may be all you need to stay dry. Sometimes, however, you may need a little more help along the path to pelvic floor health. Assistance is available in a number of unique ways that will not only augment your progress toward bladder control, but will also heighten your sense of self.

One of these unique ways is The Knack. Use it throughout your training program and afterwards. It has proven to be an indispensable bladder-control technique for many women.

THE KNACK
The Knack is especially good for women who exhibit symptoms of stress urinary incontinence, such as leaking when they cough, sneeze, or rise to a standing position.

You can do this exercise either sitting or standing, but start out by sitting as you get "the knack" of it. While sitting comfortably, feet on the ground, do a fake cough and a Quick Flick or Long Hold contraction at the same time. Do it again, four or five times. Allow yourself a short rest between coughs. Whenever you find yourself about to cough or sneeze for real, do The Knack – contract.

The Knack is one of the best things you can do to test your progress throughout your work on the plan.

You'll know the exercises are working for you when you've got The Knack. If you want to test your progress, try this when your bladder is full:

* Place a folded paper towel in your underwear between your legs. Stand with your legs apart and cough hard three or four times. If you leaked urine, trace around the damp patch on the towel with a ballpoint pen.

* Place another folded paper towel in your underwear between your legs. Stand with your legs apart, but now do a hard squeeze and lift contraction at the same time you cough hard three or four times, same as before.

Did you leak as much as you did without doing the contraction? Compare the folded paper towels.

Did you leak at all? No? Then you've got The Knack – at least for the moment. Try it the next time you're about to sneeze. Squeeze hard and lift. Still dry? Okay, try it when you go to stand up, or lift a heavy object. Still dry? You've definitely got The Knack.

Having The Knack means that you have made significant progress in controlling your incontinence. Being able to hold a contraction when you cough or sneeze will help you control stress urinary incontinence. Being able to hold a contraction will also help you control overactive-bladder contractions.

And here's something else to keep in mind. When that sense of urgency to go to the bathroom makes you fear that you won't get there in time, hold a good, strong squeeze and lift for about five seconds. Remember when you were a kid and you waited too long? The crossed legs, gripping yourself? The Knack is the adult version of holding on until you get there. It will quiet the bladder until you can get to the bathroom. More specific techniques for suppressing urges can be found earlier in this section on **Bladder Training**.

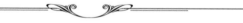

{ The Knack }

The Knack is especially useful in helping you maintain the progress you've made in controlling stress urinary incontinence. Once you've identified the specific situations, such as coughing, sneezing, getting in and out of your car, that usually caused your problem, make doing The Knack an automatic reflex whenever you do these things from now on. Practice The Knack until it becomes second nature to you. Not only will it help you maintain the strength you've developed in your pelvic floor, but it'll help prevent occasional accidents.

{ Behavior Modification }

Avoid Bladder Irritants . . . Stop Smoking . . . Check for Diabetes . . .
Reduce Emotional Stress . . . Calm Your Bladder . . .
Adopt Healthy Bowel Habits

One of the first steps in treating urinary incontinence is to eliminate any transient factors as the cause. Chief among such factors is urinary tract infections, which can trigger both stress urinary incontinence and overactive bladder. Of particular note is interstitial cystitis, a painful inflammation of the lining of the bladder that also causes urgency and frequency. As we've noted, pain is a signal that you need to see your health-care professional. If you believe that you have interstitial cystitis or you're having any pain when urinating, you're not a candidate for pelvic floor therapy until you've seen your health-care professional.

Certain classes of medications may also contribute to urinary incontinence, particularly overactive bladder. Among them are diuretics (medications that increase production of urine), sedatives, muscle relaxants, narcotics, antidepressants, drugs to control blood pressure, and even over-the-counter cough and cold remedies. (See the **Appendix** for a list of drugs and their side effects.)

When transient factors have been eliminated as a cause of your urinary incontinence, the next step is to consider your diet and daily habits. A good place to start is with your diet.

AVOID BLADDER IRRITANTS

An irritated bladder will send unnecessary and abnormal messages to your central nervous system, making you feel as if you have to urinate. Any woman with symptoms of overactive bladder knows that her bladder (*detrusor muscle*) will sometimes actually contract without her permission. By decreasing bladder irritation you will lessen the urgency and frequency of your symptoms. Bladder irritants come in many forms, and they affect individuals differently. It's important that you identify what may be irritating your bladder so you can avoid it.

Here's a list of common food and beverage irritants that should be avoided:
   ❁ Caffeine (as in coffee, tea, and certain soft drinks)
   ❁ Decaffeinated coffee (contains tannic acid, an irritant)
   ❁ Carbonation
   ❁ Aspartame and other artificial sweeteners
   ❁ Citrus fruits and juices

* Tomato products

* Vinegar

* Curry and other spicy foods

* Cantaloupe, watermelon, asparagus, and cucumber (natural diuretics)

* Alcohol (acts as a diuretic and an irritant)

Not all of the same things irritate everyone's bladder. You need to identify what irritates yours. Eliminate or significantly limit the irritants on the list for several weeks to get your bladder healthy, even those that you're sure are okay to keep. Then put a few back in your diet if you desire. You may find that your seemingly innocent cup of coffee is what's causing your bladder to misbehave. Or maybe it's that occasional craving for spicy Mexican food that worsens the problem. Once your bladder settles down again, you can reintroduce some things in moderation. Even then, you may find that certain irritants still bother your bladder, so you may have to make the sacrifice for the sake of feeling better and staying dry.

STOP SMOKING

As you know, smoking is a direct cause of many health problems, but it deserves special attention here for three reasons:

* Chronic smokers' cough exerts downward and damaging pressure on the bladder, urethra, and pelvic floor.

* Nicotine, the colorless, poisonous alkaloid to which smokers become addicted, can cause unnecessary bladder contractions and, hence, a frequent urge to urinate.

* Cigarette smokers have been shown to face an increased risk of bladder cancer.

If you have yet to find the right reason to quit, here it is. Quitting smoking may decrease the symptoms of overactive bladder. It may reduce your risk of developing stress incontinence, but will greatly reduce your chances of bladder cancer.

CHECK FOR DIABETES

The word "diabetes" stems from the Greek word meaning the discharge of excessive amounts of urine. Diabetes is any of several related metabolic disorders marked by excessive discharge of urine and persistent thirst. Early detection and treatment of diabetes can decrease the chance of developing serious complications from the disease.

Diabetes is caused by the lack of the hormone insulin or of the inability of the body to use it. Insulin is needed by the body to metabolize (to convert) sugar and starches for nutrition. A telltale sign of the disease is that diabetics tend to leak more often than non-diabetics and experience increased urgency and frequency.

REDUCE EMOTIONAL STRESS

Allow us to employ an old truism: "A woman's job is never done." In today's world, this has never been more true. Many women today are full-time working wives and mothers, selfless, well-educated "multitaskers," often expected to be the primary caregivers to small children and aged parents, full-time

{ Behavior Modification }

housekeepers and chauffeurs, and if that's not enough, lovers and intimate confidants. Some even manage to climb the corporate ladder in the meantime. Caught in the middle of a domestic pressure cooker, stressed and anxious, their health suffers. They often take care of themselves last, if at all.

Stress (even good stress such as the birth of a child), anxiety, or a bad case of nerves adversely affect the bladder by causing it to be excessively active. This causes increased symptoms of frequency and urgency. Do you remember how many trips you made to the bathroom before a big test at school or an important meeting with your boss? Stress also makes it more difficult to control or stop strong urges from turning into leaks or a rush to the bathroom.

Emotional stress is destructive. Recognizing what causes it and finding ways to reduce it may not only relieve your symptoms of overactive bladder, it may help you avoid heart disease or other diseases linked to stress. If things get to be too much for you, ask for and get help. You're a woman, yes, but you're only human.

Or it may be that you just need to learn how to relax. You've heard this before, we know, and it's easier said than done. One way to get started is to set aside five or 10 minutes a day to do nothing – not reading, not thinking about all the things you have to do – absolutely nothing. Sit in a chair, away from everyone; close your eyes and breathe deeply. Let your mind drift to pleasant thoughts. Think about your body and imagine your shoulders and your pelvis melting into the chair like butter. Imagine the space widening between your toes, your hands getting warmer. This simple meditation is therapeutic, and once you try it you'll feel surprisingly refreshed.

the
ACCIDENTAL SISTERHOOD

There are other ways to handle stress, and they work for many women: yoga, regular exercise, a walk in the woods, more sleep, and when all else fails, seek therapy.

CALM YOUR BLADDER

One of the most important things you can do to calm your bladder is to drink enough fluids. The bladder stretches as it fills and shrinks when it's empty. If you don't drink enough fluid, the functional capacity of your bladder will shrink. The less fluid you drink, the more concentrated the urine will become. Concentrated urine is more irritating to the bladder than diluted urine. It's more likely to cause inappropriate bladder contractions and more trips to the bathroom. It also encourages the growth of bacteria, which may lead to infections that can cause incontinence.

Drinking too much fluid can be a problem, too. We see women every day clutching a bottle of water wherever they go. Evidently, they believe they have to drink at least two quarts of water every day, in addition to the coffee, tea, juice or whatever else they may drink in the course of the day. Running all that fluid through your system would make anybody have to go a lot.

We recommend drinking a total of six to eight eight-ounce glasses of non-bladder-irritating fluids daily – remembering to avoid the common bladder irritants in the list we gave. It's best to drink fluids in small servings. And take the fluid from fruits and vegetables into account as part of your daily total.

ADOPT HEALTHY BOWEL HABITS

Constipation is a major factor in female bladder control and urinary incontinence. A rectum that is full of waste (stool) presses against and irritates the bladder, which can't hold a normal volume of urine. The result is an increase in the urgency and frequency of urination – the symptoms of overactive bladder.

Constipation may also aggravate the symptoms of stress urinary incontinence. With a full bowel already pressing on the bladder, the amount of intra-abdominal pressure needed to cause a leak when you cough or sneeze will be less.

It's important to relieve constipation and regain regular bowel movements. A full discussion of the steps you can take to improve bowel habits can be found in **Healthy Bowel Function** in the **Appendix**, along with **Fiber Facts**, a list of foods high in fiber, which can be helpful.

Please take careful note: We strenuously recommend that anyone who sees blood in her stool or has chronic constipation should see a health-care professional. Blood in the stool can be a symptom of a serious, possibly life-threatening condition.

{ Commitment for Life }

Feel It Forever

Your most difficult and demanding task lies ahead. It's staying with the program, not just for a while until you've worked your way safely out the woods. The hot breath of complacency will never be far behind. So be alert: when you reach the point where you're getting through each day confidently dry, when life in the bedroom is better than ever, and when you think that you can stop exercising – don't. The only way to keep the strength and stamina of any of your body's voluntary muscles – your arms, your legs, your abdomen, your back and shoulders, your pelvic floor – all that you worked so hard to achieve – is to exercise them regularly. Keep focused on maintaining your results.

Typically, to maintain your pelvic floor strength, we recommend that you do all the exercises in your Personal Progressive Exercise Log at least three times a week. In addition, do a few Long Holds and Quick Flicks every day. This is enough to keep most women dry or at their current pelvic floor fitness level. If you find yourself falling off the exercise bandwagon, resume your daily exercise to get back on board.

Once you're where you need to be, you can maintain the holding tone and reflex strength of your pelvic floor muscles — exercising both types of muscle contractions, short and long, Long Holds and Quick Flicks — by doing them throughout the day.

Make doing the exercises a habit. Use these handy cues as reminders to do your pelvic floor exercises:

- Every time you change the baby or wash your hands.
- When you're in the car and stopped at a red light.
- When you're waiting at a retail counter to pay for a purchase.
- When you're among friends at a party with a cool drink in your hand.
- When you're sitting and watching television.
- And don't forget to practice The Knack.

You get the idea. Will anyone else know what you're doing? Not unless you tell them. But they might ask you why you're smiling.

Another thing, find yourself an "Accountability Partner." This is a fancy way of saying having someone involved in The Sisterhood Plan you can trust to help you stay on the path of pelvic floor health and fitness. This may be another member of the Sisterhood, your partner, or a close friend who will step off the sidelines to encourage and support you.

Get this person to . . .

* Ask you how you're doing from time to time.

* Ask you if you're remembering to do your exercises.

* Raise his or her eyebrows when you reach for the coffeepot.

* Say, "C'mon, you don't have to go 'just in case.' We won't be away that long," when he or she sees you heading for the bathroom.

Perhaps you can persuade your Accountability Partner to join you on the path, where you can encourage each other. (Men can benefit, too.) It's healthy to get it out in the open, and it's a good way to stay informed and find out what other women are thinking and saying about it.

Talk to a friend about the problem. We know it won't be easy, but by opening up to another woman you may find that you've helped her understand her problem and encouraged her to seek help for it. Tell her about The Sisterhood Plan, direct her to our Web site, and recommend a health-care professional who can help her overcome her problem. Show her the way to a better quality of life, free from emotionally crippling bladder and pelvic floor issues. That's what friends are for.

By continuing to exercise, modifying your diet, and rethinking your bathroom habits, you'll be empowered to change your life. By being there for other women who suffer from similar issues, you can actually make a difference in other women's lives.

Commit to yourself. Commit to each other.

And remember: don't stop smiling. Ever.

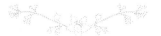

DEVICES . . . AND DESIRE

{ Devices: There's Help Where You Need It }
Getting Wired . . . Getting Feedback . . . Weight Training

GETTING WIRED

The last thing we want to see happen is for you to try to exercise your pelvic floor muscles and not quite get the hang of it.

What we want to see happen is for you to do the exercises and get results.

The truth is, though, sometimes we all need a little help getting started on something that, up until now, we haven't given much thought to. The pelvic floor muscles are that "something" for many women. Fortunately, there are a number of therapeutic devices that will help you get over your initial hurdles and on your way to pelvic floor health.

Not being able to feel or contract your pelvic floor muscles is the highest hurdle. The muscles may be too weak to respond.

What's more, the signals that you're trying to send to them may not be getting there because injury or long disuse may have deadened the nerves. This is not as serious as it may seem. New muscle fibers can be recruited and the pelvic floor may be re-innervated or stimulated.

Enlivening the muscles of the pelvic floor is possible in the same way that muscles of the legs or arms can be rehabilitated. In the case of the large muscles of a leg, for example, a therapist will move the leg, simulating the normal contraction and relaxation of the muscles. Over time, this simple act of having someone else assist in moving a leg that won't move on its own will awaken and recruit new muscle fibers. Gradually, the ability to move the leg will return and the muscles will get stronger as the therapist continues to exercise them with you.

Obviously, the muscles of the pelvic floor can't be exercised in the same way that a person's leg can be. So another way to reach them had to be found. That way is through electrical impulses, and a physical therapist trained in pelvic floor therapy is your access to this technological approach. Electrical stimulation, or E-stim, is a *controlled delivery of very small amounts* of electrical stimulation to the muscles of the pelvic floor. The pulsed electrical stimulation causes the muscles to contract and relax, much like the way our nerves make our muscles contract and relax. It's used to help a person beginning the exercises strengthen very weak muscles and is usually delivered through a tampon-like device placed in the vagina or rectum.

Electrical stimulation has also been shown to decrease the over-activity of the bladder. The stimulated contraction of the pelvic floor muscles signals the bladder to reduce its contractions. This mimics what happens when you're able to contract your pelvic floor muscles to reduce the urge to urinate.

Additionally, some studies have also shown that electrical stimulation can also assist in strengthening the pelvic floor muscles by helping to realign the muscle fibers. This effect particularly improves the ability of an incontinent woman to strengthen her fast-twitch contractions to stop sudden leaks when she coughs or sneezes.

There's a more ambitious device that delivers electrical stimulation to a patient while she sits fully clothed on a comfortable chair. According to the manufacturer, the NeoControl® Pelvic Floor Therapy System stimulates more of the muscles in the pelvic floor than the systems that use vaginal or rectal probes. The company also claims that "patients treated with NeoControl have reported significant improvements in their quality of life." One may take this to mean a number of things.

The NeoControl company calls the technology behind the chair Extracorporeal Magnetic Innervation, or ExMI™ for short. No active participation by the patient is required. She sits in the chair as the magnetic pulses are aimed at the muscles of the pelvic floor. The pelvic floor muscles contract and relax with each pulse. Since the patient does not actively engage the muscles herself, she may see her symptoms return when she stops using the chair. But the chair therapy may help a patient learn how to contract and exercise her pelvic floor muscles. It may also innervate or realign the muscle fibers to the point where a patient can begin to exercise them herself. It appears to us that if a patient combines pelvic muscle training with her sessions on the chair, she could achieve long-term benefits.

GETTING FEEDBACK

Biofeedback is a treatment technique in which people are trained to improve their health by using signals from their own bodies. Simply put, when you step on a bathroom scale or take your temperature, you're using biofeedback. The scale tells you if you've gained or lost weight, and your response might be to change your diet. If an oral thermometer tells you that you have a fever, your response might be to rest and drink plenty of fluids.

Because you can't see the pelvic muscles you're working on or how they're improving, biofeedback (Dr. Kegel's contribution to pelvic floor therapy) is a way for you to know if you're exercising the correct muscles and how well you're doing it.

Biofeedback for pelvic floor therapy is usually performed in the office by a physical therapist or a nurse specialist. A small sensor is placed either in the vagina, the anus, or just outside one or the other. Additional sensors may be placed on the abdomen or buttocks. The procedure is painless. It can be a necessary and important step for many women beginning pelvic floor therapy.

The sensors measure the small electrical signals that all muscles produce when they contract. The sensors are connected to a computer that displays the incoming electrical signals on a monitor. The patient can then see if she's contracting the proper set of muscles and how strongly she's doing it. The computer will store the information from each session, allowing the patient to see her progress as her pelvic floor muscles get stronger.

WEIGHT TRAINING

Centuries ago in China, some say Japan, women learned to treat themselves with three small balls inserted in their vaginas. Made of wood or jade, sometimes hollow with smaller metal balls or even mercury inside, they were strung together by a fine metal chain, and had a silk cord at one end for retrieval. Known today as *ben wa* balls, they may have been one of the first devices for pelvic floor muscle training. Today, we have vaginal weights for that purpose. Contracting the pelvic floor muscles keeps the weight in place, keeping it from falling out.

Vaginal weights help women identify and exercise specific muscle groups in the pelvic floor. They are available as single-weighted devices or as systems of progressively heavier weights ranging from a few ounces to a half pound. We recommend the progressive weight system. It allows you to challenge yourself progressively as your muscles get stronger. Some women, however, need help getting started with the weights. A physical therapist can offer that help, and more.

The principle of progressive vaginal weights is based on the same principle used to train other muscles of the body. For instance, you exercise your bicep muscles every time you bend your arms. They'll get stronger if you start exercising with five-pound dumbbells and then progress to 10-, 15-, or 20-pound weights. The same thing goes for your pelvic floor. But you'll be using weights measured in ounces, not pounds. Progressive weight training will increase the strength of your pelvic floor muscles, improve your symptoms and, not to be overlooked, heighten your sexual response.

Some women find that they can reach their goals without the assistance of vaginal weights; others find that they accelerate their therapy. The weights may also provide a kind of feedback or sensation they find useful when doing their pelvic floor exercises. The wearer can feel herself squeezing around the weight and recognizes that she's doing the exercise correctly. This also gives her a sense of how strong her squeeze is getting to be.

Two such progressive systems are marketed: Femtone™ and StepFree™. Femtone consists of a set of five vaginal cones of varying weights made from surgical-grade stainless steel. Each one is encased in a double-welded plastic cone with a plastic-coated retrieval cord.

The other brand of weights – the StepFree vaginal weight system – offers five different-sized weights that fit into a two-piece plastic cone, which also has a retrieval cord. Exchanging a heavier weight for a lighter one in the plastic cone can gradually increase resistance.

When the cone of either brand is inserted into the vagina, the pelvic floor muscles must contract to keep it in place. Sensing that the cone is slipping out of her, the wearer will contract her pelvic floor muscles to hold it in. In doing so, she's more likely to be using the correct muscles. The cone provides a variable amount of resistance depending on which of the weights you're using at the time. You can keep the cone inside you while doing various activities, especially your pelvic floor exercises. When you can hold it in for longer than 15 minutes, you may try coughing, climbing stairs, or jogging in place.

Used properly along with the pelvic floor exercises, the vaginal cones will help increase pelvic muscle strength and improve your symptoms of bladder urgency and incontinence. At that point, you can just use them a few times a week or whenever you feel you're losing some of the benefit you've gained from them.

In addition to the cones, you may wish to explore single-weight vaginal resistive devices. One such device is the FPT – Feminine Personal Trainer. Shaped like an hourglass (three and half inches long), one rounded ball-like end is larger than the other. It's made of surgical-grade stainless steel and is available in two sizes: 12 ounces and 16 ounces. One end, usually the larger, is inserted in the vagina. The user contracts her pelvic floor muscles to hold it in place while she does a series of pelvic floor contractions. The FPT's shape permits a woman to use either end of the device. The smaller end would require a stronger pelvic floor contraction to keep it in place, as would either end of the heavier version, which might be daunting for some women.

Resistance training weights like the FPT, while interesting and probably helpful, do not provide the gradient weight training that we prefer. They are often promoted for their erotic potential, and if that's what it takes to get you to exercise your pelvic floor, then that's fine. It all contributes to the same cause – a healthy pelvic floor.

Which system of weights is for you? As we said, we like the vaginal cones. But you may wish to experiment with other approaches.

A truism has it that "there's nothing new under the sun." Vaginal weights and *ben wa* balls? Maybe just a new wrinkle to a very old custom.

{ Desire: The Power of The Secret Squeeze }
Sexual Disorder . . . Sexual Response

"Love is the irresistible desire to be irresistibly desired."
— Robert Frost —

The muscles of the pelvic floor are an integral part of the orgasmic mechanism. At the moment of climax, the muscles contract in rhythmic waves creating the pulsating nature of the orgasm. The stronger the muscles, the stronger the orgasm.

For a woman with bladder-control issues, desire is often accompanied by "avoid." (Sorry pun intended.) But avoid what? You don't need it spelled out for you. And you know why: the unexpected leaking and embarrassment, the feeling of a need to urinate during intercourse, the pelvic organ bulging into the vagina and its discomfort. A woman who finds herself in any of these situations may have lost something very dear to her:

the
ACCIDENTAL SISTERHOOD

spontaneity – the freedom to abandon herself to the pleasure of sexual intimacy without anxiety.

The Sisterhood Plan is a proven first line of therapy for the treatment of bladder-control issues. It will help you overcome symptoms of overactive bladder and stress urinary incontinence, the issues that usually cause urine leakage during sex. Occasionally, merely emptying your bladder beforehand may be all you need to do. But the problem for some women may be more complex.

Following childbirth or pelvic surgery, a woman may find to her dismay that she sometimes doesn't reach an orgasm in sexual intercourse and, when she does, that it's weaker than it used to be. She knows it's not right, but she soldiers on, often beset by depression and an increasingly frustrated partner. A blunted sexual response threatens a woman's belief in her femininity and her power to arouse. She's lost something very dear to her and probably feels helpless to do anything about it.

Sexual dysfunctions can be lifelong problems. They can show up only in certain situations, or develop after a period of normal sexual function, such as we've just described. The causes can be psychological, physical, or both.

Psychological causes can include:
- ❁ Conflicts with a partner
- ❁ Worry about sexual performance
- ❁ Self-esteem
- ❁ Stress or anxiety

❈ Depression

❈ History of rape or sexual abuse

Physical causes can include:

❈ Disease (such as diabetes or heart disease)

❈ Pelvic surgery, injury, or trauma

❈ Alcohol or drug abuse

❈ Medication side effects

❈ Hormone deficiency

❈ Neurological disorders

Sex therapy is often recommended for sexual dysfunctions that stem from psychological or relationship issues. On the other hand, problems resulting from physical causes respond to medical treatment and physical therapy. When physical causes are resolved, it may help you overcome accompanying emotional issues. If not, see a therapist.

Sex Shouldn't Be Painful

The first thing any woman experiencing pain during sexual intercourse should do is to see a health-care professional. Pain is your body's way of telling you that something is wrong. Please, don't ignore it; there's no reason why a health-care professional skilled in the treatment of female pelvic floor disorders can't help you.

Vaginal dryness can be the cause of the pain. It often occurs during and after menopause and is easily remedied with personal lubricants. Your gynecologist may also recommend or prescribe estrogen creams or insertable tablets. A urinary tract infection may be responsible for the pain, as will interstitial cystitis, an inflammation of the lining of the bladder. A seriously prolapsed organ will sometimes be uncomfortable to a woman during sex. A mild prolapse doesn't have to interfere with sexual intercourse. Any discomfort from penetration will lessen as the muscles surrounding the vagina are better able to support the pelvic organs and restore a smoother, less obstructed path.

Another cause of pain is vaginal tightness, or *vaginismus*. This condition is the involuntary spasm or constant tension of the muscles surrounding the opening of the vagina. Anything entering the vagina will cause pain. Exercise therapy can help. By exercising the muscles of the pelvic floor, they become more flexible, as well as stronger. Intercourse will be less uncomfortable as the exercises are continued.

Some women also find that, as they age, the walls of their vaginas atrophy, or grow thinner. Sex becomes uncomfortable and, over time, may be avoided. Pelvic floor exercises can help rebuild the vaginal walls. In the meantime, personal lubricants are useful as a woman improves the tone and condition of her pelvic floor.

Orgasm and Desire

The problems associated with orgasm and desire, however, are more complex. Apart from someone who has undergone female genital mutilation or female circumcision (the cutting off of a girl's clitoral bud or glans, which is practiced in some cultures) most women are able to experience orgasm. Some women, it's true, with normal genitalia have never had an orgasm. That's said to be about 10 percent of women. But this may have more to do with them and their partners not knowing how the female body responds to sexual stimulation than to anything else.

It used to be said that a woman who rarely or never experienced orgasm was *anorgasmic*. The term is dismissive, in that it suggests that the woman is not capable of having an orgasm, or that she was "frigid" and not capable of enjoying a normal sexual response. Neither term is appropriate and both are woefully out of date. Their use over the years may have had something to do with the myth of the vaginal orgasm.

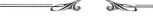

{ *The Origin of the Vibrator* }

In the late 19th and early 20th century, on the strength of the questionable notion of vaginal orgasm, sexually frustrated women were led to believe that their problem was psychological. Bizarre as it now seems, the treatment for this "psychological" problem was to have their vulvas massaged . . . by a doctor. The patient's response was described in the medical literature as a "paroxysm." It isn't surprising that it afforded these women some measure of relief. Evidently, the doctors knew something they weren't sharing with their patients − or their patients' husbands − that stimulation of the vagina alone normally doesn't lead to orgasm. Incidentally, the practice of vulva (clitoral) massage led to the invention of the vibrator − about 10 years before the vacuum cleaner.

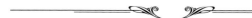

It's exceptionally rare for a woman with a healthy clitoris to be truly anorgasmic. Today, it's more appropriate to say that a sexually active woman who seldom or never reaches an orgasm is *preorgasmic*. That is to say, simply, that she just hasn't had an orgasm . . . yet, or at least regularly.

As with overactive bladder, the problem of the absent or weak orgasm can have a transient or external cause. Drug treatment for certain conditions, such as depression and hypothyroidism, and even high blood pressure, can lower sexual desire and interfere with orgasm. That's for a woman and her health-care professional to determine.

It's not our intention here to offer advice on overcoming an array of sexual problems; for that we refer you to a qualified sex therapist, or any number of sexuality guides, such as the few we've included in our list of references in the back of this book. The guides offer information that can help people understand what's happening in their relationships and where, if necessary, they can find help, especially from a professional skilled in counseling individuals and couples. Our purpose is to restore and preserve the health and fitness of your pelvic floor in order to alleviate and cure the symptoms of urgency and urinary incontinence, which offers sexual benefits as well.

In our experience, setting aside external physical and emotional factors, when we improve anatomical understanding, what we see is that a woman with a healthy pelvic floor can enjoy optimal sexual satisfaction. The Sisterhood Plan, particularly through its regimen of exercises, pays a substantial sexual dividend. A healthy and strengthened pelvic floor is vital to you if you want to enjoy good sex with a loving and considerate partner.

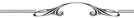

{ Get A Grip }

A woman's strong and healthy pelvic floor also plays a major role in pleasuring her partner. In fact, penis size shouldn't matter to a woman with a strong pelvic floor; she can contract to grip and squeeze whatever he has to offer. Both participants benefit. And she is further empowered by heightening the pleasure of her partner. Not every woman's sexual partner has a penis, and that's a fact. It's just that those partners who do have penises tend to be the more likely secondary *beneficiaries of a woman's strong pelvic floor. The* primary *beneficiary is, in any case, the woman.*

{ The PC Muscle }

One of the specific muscles that provide the "contractions" of the vagina is known as the PC muscle. You may have read or heard about the PC muscle. PC stands for pubucoccygeus, which is the anatomical name of one of the pelvic floor muscles. It wraps around the vagina and, when contracted, squeezes the vagina. It's often mentioned in the context of Kegel exercises to enhance vaginal intercourse.

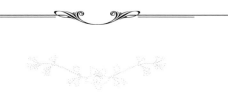

A Promise to Keep

The Accidental Sisterhood Progressive Plan is a response to an enormous problem facing many women – a problem that is too often ignored and vastly underestimated. We believe that every woman can benefit from it . . . that *you* can benefit from it.

You have in your possession a unique way to correct or prevent problems arising from disorders of the pelvic floor. It is a *detailed* and *doable* plan to regain control of your bladder and your life.

This book is about healing and strengthening your pelvic floor – everything about it, not just the symptoms of incontinence or urgency. This book is about *you* regaining authority over a fundamental part of *your* body that you might otherwise have felt was beyond your control.

You found that you *can* learn to make your bladder behave. You *can* control the muscles of your pelvic floor to improve or cure urinary incontinence and urgency. You *can* make your sex life better.

For the vast majority of women who must struggle every day with these issues, The Sisterhood Plan will not only free them from urgency and wetting, it will, like coming upon an unexpected treasure, strengthen their physical response to sex.

Women have always had to work harder, often on their own, to get where they wanted to be. And when they got there, they knew it *wasn't* by accident.

But we don't expect you to go it all alone. We're here for you. We'll work with you for as long as you need us – for more information, for encouragement, for help.

Contact us through our Web site, *www.AccidentalSisterhood.com*. We want to know how you've done on The Sisterhood Plan and what you think about it. Tell us how we can improve our program, how we might help others.

You can help, too, as we've already suggested. Share your knowledge with others. Talk to other women about these issues and, yes, even how you've learned to master yours. Tell your best friend, your mother. Tell your daughter. Above all, tell your sisters . . . *The Accidental Sisterhood.*

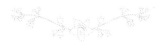

A PROMISE TO KEEP

BEYOND PELVIC FLOOR THERAPY

{ Getting to the Bottom of Your Problem }
A Guide to Diagnosis

Seeking a diagnosis is the first step in treating incontinence and achieving bladder freedom. The best place to start is your health-care professional, who may be an internist, a general practitioner, or, for many women, a gynecologist, a nurse practitioner, or physician's assistant. If your health-care professional is not experienced in treating incontinence, or if you'd like a second opinion, you may want to see a specialist. Gynecologists and urologists are likely to have more experience treating incontinence. There may be a continence clinic or specialist in female pelvic medicine in your area. This health-care professional may be a urologist or a gynecologist who did a fellowship (extra training) in female pelvic medicine and reconstructive surgery.

Ask your health-care professional for a referral or call a

university medical center, hospital, or medical society. In most cases, a health-care professional's initial diagnosis will determine if your symptoms indicate one of the most common problems: overactive bladder, stress incontinence, or a combination of both problems.

For the names of health-care professionals and other information, visit the American Urogynecologic Society (AUS) Web site, *www.augs.org*, and the American Urological Association (AUA) Web sites: *www.auanet.org* (general information about AUA) and *www.urologyhealth.org* (AUA's online patient information resource).

Prepare to make the most of your appointment. Keep a record of when you go to the bathroom and when you have leakage for at least two days before you see the health-care professional. Your Voiding Diary is perfect for this purpose. Note whether an activity such as sneezing, lifting, standing up, or sex seems to bring on leakage, or whether it occurs suddenly and without warning. Record the time of day or night when the incidents take place. Write down what you eat and drink each day, but don't change your habits just yet; you need to know what is really happening. Make a list of your medicines, including any over-the-counter drugs that you take occasionally, and bring it to the appointment.

Make a list of questions for the health-care professional before your appointment, such as:

- ❀ Why am I having this problem? Is it overactive bladder, urge incontinence, or stress urinary incontinence?
- ❀ Do you see many people with problems like this?

{ Getting to the Bottom of Your Problem }

❀ Do I have other health problems that may be contributing to it?

❀ Can the condition be treated? How?

❀ What are the likely outcomes of these treatments?

❀ Is surgery ever necessary for this condition?

❀ Is there anything I can do for myself to improve the problem?

❀ Should I see a specialist for this condition?

Be sure that you understand the answers before you leave the office. If you don't feel the health-care professional is concerned with finding a cause, or hasn't had significant experience treating other people with the problem, see another health-care professional. While great strides have recently been made in understanding and treating incontinence, not all doctors have the same degree of familiarity with the condition. You need to find one who has experience and up-to-date knowledge.

Be candid and exact about your condition with the health-care professional. You may find it embarrassing to discuss your urinary problem, but the health-care professional will understand if you have difficulty talking about the condition. Describing your symptoms is an important part of the examination, so explain what you mean in detail, being as specific as possible. For some people, "leaking a lot" might mean they feel damp; for others, it might mean a flood. Explain clearly what is happening to you.

Be willing to answer questions about your lifestyle (eating, drinking, sleeping, exercise, and sexual activity) and your emotional situation as it relates to your symptoms. Having your leakage record with you will help you to help the health-care professional. Because incontinence involves the urinary system, as well as the nervous system and pelvic muscles, your health-care professional will usually do abdominal, rectal, pelvic, and neurological examinations. Your examination will be similar to your yearly PAP smear.

The health-care professional may wish to do additional tests, such as asking you to cough while lying down and standing up, and to bend, bounce, or walk. These actions test for stress urinary incontinence, which is the most common type of incontinence.

You should be asked for a urine sample to check for abnormalities or infection. After you have urinated, the health-care professional may check to see if your bladder emptied completely by doing a bladder catheterization or ultrasound. For a catheterization, a sterile tube is passed through your urethra into the bladder to drain any remaining urine. This procedure can be uncomfortable, but it isn't painful.

Another test that might be done in the office is to insert a long-handled cotton swab into the urethra to see if the urethra has dropped out of normal position. Sometimes the health-care professional may also order blood tests to check how well your kidneys are working.

Based on your history, the interview, your leakage record, and these tests, the health-care professional may be able to prescribe treatment. However, if more information is needed to make a diagnosis, the doctor might order additional tests. Some women may find these tests embarrassing because a typical examination involves examination of their genitals and, in some cases, requires trying to get a patient to leak while someone else is watching. Nevertheless, these tests can be crucial in identifying an underlying cause of the incontinence or bladder problem.

At the conclusion of the initial visit — or follow-up appointment if additional testing is required — you should have an understanding of the type of bladder problem, or incontinence problem, you are having and what treatment options are available to you. You should have both a conservative and/or a surgical treatment option. Or, as is often the case, you may elect to try a conservative route of therapy first or move on with further testing before any decision is made.

Depending on your health-care professional's initial examination, he or she may recommend additional tests. A number of tests are useful in diagnosing bladder problems. Chief among them is a series of tests referred to as "urodynamics," which is designed to determine how a patient's bladder works at several levels.

Urodynamics includes the following tests:

❀ *Uroflowmetry — measures how rapidly the bladder empties.* With a full bladder, you urinate into a collecting device attached to a computer. The instrument determines how long it takes for the stream to start, the amount voided each second, the strength and smoothness of the stream, and any dripping after urination. There is no discomfort.

❀ *Cystometry — measures the pressure in the bladder as it fills.* A catheter is inserted through the urethra into the bladder, and the bladder is then filled with sterile water. A second catheter is placed in the vagina to measure increases in abdominal pressure. You signal when you feel the bladder filling and when you feel you must urinate. During the study, and when your bladder is full, you will be asked to cough and bear down to see if leakage occurs. At the conclusion of the study, you will be asked to empty your bladder with the catheter still in place. This is very helpful in understanding how your bladder works. The procedure should not be painful, though there may be discomfort from the catheter. Cystometry has a number of goals:

~ To understand how well your bladder holds urine.

~ To see if the bladder contracts when it should not (overactive bladder).

~ To see at what pressure you leak.

~ To understand how tight a seal the urethra makes.

~ To understand how well the bladder squeezes when you empty and if the sphincter and pelvic muscles work together.

❀ *Urethral pressure profile – measures pressure in the urethra and compares it with bladder pressure.* A catheter is passed through the urethra into the bladder; the bladder is filled with about three ounces of water, and bladder pressure is measured. Then the catheter is slowly pulled back through the urethra, measuring pressure at different points. The test may be repeated while you cough or bear down. Again, there may be mild discomfort from the catheter.

❀ *Pressure flow – measures how well the sphincter and bladder are coordinated and how well the bladder functions during emptying.* Typically, this test is done at the conclusion of the above studies and involves emptying your bladder with the catheter still in place.

Urodynamics may be done with or without X-rays, and video technology can also be used to observe bladder and urethral functions.

Other tests that might also be used include:

Cystoscopy provides an inside view of the urethra and bladder by passing a narrow tube, called a cystoscope, through the urethra into the bladder. When the cystoscope is in place, the bladder is filled with a sterile solution. This test may be mildly uncomfortable. It's performed in the office with the use of a numbing gel.

Voiding Cystourethrography uses X-rays to examine the bladder and urethra. The test includes an X-ray of the abdomen and pelvis to determine the position of kidneys, ureters, and bladder. It also checks for abnormalities of the spine, any abnormal masses, bowel impaction, or kidney stones. Then a catheter is passed through the urethra into the bladder and the bladder is filled with liquid that is visible on an X-ray film. X-rays of the bladder are taken from several angles. Finally, you are asked to bear down and finally urinate while X-rays are taken of the urethra. After urination, another X-ray is taken to check for liquid remaining in the bladder. There may be mild discomfort from the catheter.

Ultrasound may also be used to check the shape, size, and location of the kidneys, ureters, and bladder. It's also used to find out how much urine the bladder holds. There is no discomfort.

As you can see, a full spectrum of tests is available to enable your health-care professional to establish a firm diagnosis of your bladder and incontinence problem. It is very likely that you would undergo some or most of these tests in the course of your examination.

the
ACCIDENTAL SISTERHOOD

BEYOND PELVIC FLOOR THERAPY

{ Drug Therapy }

An Expanding Option for Overactive Bladder

Medications to treat urinary incontinence are directed at the bladder and are used to treat the urgency, frequency, and urge-incontinence symptoms of overactive bladder. None, however, is specifically available for stress urinary incontinence.

Patients frequently ask these two questions: "Why does this problem develop?" and "How do the medications work?" Unfortunately, our answer to the first question isn't very helpful: No one knows precisely why some people develop an overactive bladder. We know that certain things irritate the bladder and, once eliminated, the bladder behaves better. We also know that an overactive-bladder problem is connected to nerve and muscle changes. Certain events seem to be related to these changes. These include aging, recurrent urinary tract infections, pregnancy, vaginal and caesarian delivery, pelvic or vaginal surgery of any type (hysterectomy, bladder surgery), radiation therapy for cancer, and other reasons unknown to us.

How the medications work, however, is clear to us: drugs to treat overactive bladder belong to a class of drugs known as anticholinergics, which decrease nerve impulses and, thereby, reduce spasms of smooth muscle, such as the bladder. The drugs have several effects: they reduce the strength and frequency of bladder contractions, or urges to urinate, and delay, but may not eliminate, urges.

Medications can be used in two ways. Some people find that taking a medication for overactive bladder is a simple solution to their problem. If it improves their symptoms with minimal side effects, they may continue it for life. Note that medication does not cure the problem; it only controls it. If stopped, the symptoms will return.

Another approach to medication therapy is to start medication at the same time that you begin strengthening your pelvic floor. Once you have developed bladder control you can decrease or stop the medication.

PRESCRIPTION MEDICATIONS USED TO TREAT OVERACTIVE BLADDER		
GENERIC NAME	BRAND NAME	DRUG ACTION
Darifenicin	Enablex®	Decreases bladder contractions and increases bladder capacity.
Oxybutynin	Ditropan®	
Oxybutynin extended release	Ditropan®XL	
Oxybutynin transdermal	Oxytrol®	
Solifenacin Succinate	VESIcare®	
Tolterodine	Detrol®	
Tolterodine extended release	Detrol®LA	
Trospium chloride	SANCTURA®	

Some key points to keep in mind about bladder medications:

❀ Bladder medications increase the amount of urine the bladder can hold before it gives the signal to urinate. Also, if the bladder starts contracting, or squeezing, when you don't want it to, the medications can reduce the strength of the contraction so you don't leak.

❀ The most common complaints from patients taking the medications are dry mouth, blurry vision, constipation, and skin flushing. Some patients, usually older but not necessarily, may develop some confusion from the medications.

❀ The drugs are generally well tolerated. However, all patients are different and respond differently to medications. It's never clear why some patients respond and some do not, nor is it understood why some patients are sensitive to a particular medication and experience side effects.

❀ You should not take medicines for overactive bladder if

you have an eye problem known as uncontrolled narrow-angle glaucoma, or if your stomach empties slowly, or if you have trouble emptying your bladder. Urinary retention (incomplete bladder emptying) is usually evaluated on your first doctor visit by ultrasound or by passing a small catheter into the bladder to check how much urine is left in your bladder after you urinate.

❀ It is always advisable to check with your health-care professional before taking any medications if you are pregnant, trying to become pregnant, or breast-feeding.

❀ There are no clear data that one medication is better than another medication. While the medications are primarily indicated for patients with overactive bladder-wet and overactive bladder-dry, every now and then a patient with stress incontinence will experience significant improvement with the medication.

❀ Many patients say that they can't use a bladder medication because they have kidney problems or are on a water pill. This is not true. These medications only affect the bladder; they have no effect on kidney function.

❀ After you start a medication, it takes a minimum of two to six weeks to see a change in urgency or frequency.

❀ The medications will work better if you add The Sisterhood Plan's behavioral recommendations and our Progressive Pelvic Floor Exercises to your treatment program.

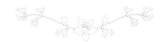

{ Surgery and Other Options for Overactive Bladder, Stress Urinary Incontinence, and Prolapse }

Correcting Overactive Bladder . . . Correcting Stress Urinary Incontinence . . . Correcting Prolapse . . . Postscript to Surgery and Staying Dry for Good

Improvements in the surgical treatment of urinary incontinence, as well as pelvic organ prolapse, have progressed dramatically over the last decade. For any one patient, the approach that would be the most appropriate for her depends on the evaluation of her condition and what she elects to do. The information that you will find in this section will, in considerable detail, describe the surgical choices, as well as the use of the pessary, a non-surgical option. Incontinence is not life threatening; you don't have to do anything about it if you don't want to. But, of course, you know and we know that that's not really an option for most, if not all, women who live with this problem.

{ Surgery Outcomes Are Encouraging }
Eighty-five percent of patients will be dry after surgery and 95 percent will be dry or significantly improved. While your chances of a cure are very high, not every case of urinary incontinence will be cured. Neither pelvic floor therapy nor surgery may be appropriate in every case. And a few patients will fail to respond at all.

While we can't back it up with any substantive data today, our experience suggests – and we hope to demonstrate – that surgical outcomes are better for patients who have first improved the condition of their bladder and pelvic floor muscles through pelvic floor therapy. Understanding and practicing our Behavior Modification program, particularly, can pay a high dividend after surgery.

Once the patient elects to proceed with surgery, we follow a specific protocol:

- ❀ First, we determine the patient's worst bladder symptoms – stress urinary incontinence, overactive bladder-wet, overactive bladder-dry, or both.

- ❀ If the patient presents symptoms of both overactive bladder and stress urinary incontinence, we usually correct the overactive bladder symptoms first. That's because overactive bladder tends to be the most challenging, or the most unpredictable, for the patient.

- ❀ Finally, we correct the stress incontinence symptoms when the overactive bladder symptoms have been improved.

CORRECTING OVERACTIVE BLADDER

Among the surgical procedures developed to treat overactive bladder, one, in particular, uses "pacemaker" implant technology to regulate bladder function:

S3 Neuromodulation – InterStim®

The Medtronic InterStim® System for Urinary Control is indicated for the treatment of the symptoms of overactive bladder, including overactive bladder-wet (or urinary urge incontinence), significant symptoms of overactive bladder-dry (or urgency-frequency), and urinary retention.

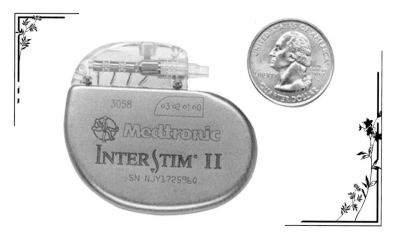

InterStim Therapy uses a thin, small-diameter, battery-operated device to send mild electrical pulses to a nerve located in the lower back (just above the tailbone). This nerve, called the sacral nerve, influences the bladder and surrounding muscles that manage the urinary function. The electrical stimulation may eliminate or reduce certain bladder-control symptoms in some people. The system is surgically placed under the skin.

The implantation procedure uses a tined lead – a thin electrical wire prong – that is placed near the sacral nerve. The procedure typically takes less than an hour and requires two small incisions on the upper surface of the buttock.

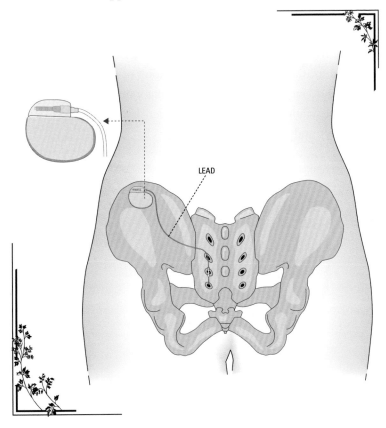

LEAD

❋ The neural stimulator sends a constant signal to the nerve that controls the bladder; it quiets the urge and restores normal control of the need to urinate.

❋ The implant doesn't need to be turned on and off.

{ Surgery and Other Options for Overactive Bladder,
Stress Urinary Incontinence, and Prolapse }

❋ The procedure is done in two outpatient sessions and requires mild sedation and local anesthesia; you don't need to go to sleep.

❋ At the first session, the nerve is located and the wire, or lead, is positioned near the nerve. An *external* neural stimulator is used at first to evaluate the patient's response during a two-week testing stage. The external neural stimulator is about the size of a cell phone and clips at the waist in the same fashion. The power supply of the stimulator is left on at all times, except when showering. During the testing period the patient is asked to keep a diary to evaluate the effectiveness of the therapy.

❋ At the second session, two to three weeks later, if the procedure is working for the patient, a stimulator – much smaller than the test stimulator – is implanted under the skin. The external stimulator is no longer needed.

❋ Patients who have had a successful testing stage have a 90 percent chance of doing well with the implant.

❋ Battery life of the implanted stimulator is from three to 10 years, depending on the model.

❋ There have been no reports of nerve injury, but as in any invasive technique, there is a risk of infection.

❋ InterStim Therapy is covered by most insurance plans, including Medicare.

❋ InterStim Therapy was first approved by the U.S. Food and Drug Administration in 1997. Medtronic, the manufacturer, was granted approval for a newer, less invasive method in 2002 that is encouraging wider use of the procedure.

❋ New applications of neuromodulation continue to evolve, such as for bowel dysfunction currently under investigation in Europe.

Botox®

Botox (botulinum toxin type A) injections, most widely known for temporarily smoothing out frown lines between the eyebrows, have been shown to relax the bladder and reduce the urge to urinate. This is a new use for botulinum toxin and not yet covered by insurance plans. Early research appears promising. Some questions raised about its use in treating overactive bladder include:

❀ How much of the drug should be injected into the bladder?

❀ How often are the injections needed?

❀ Will the procedure be covered by patients' health insurance?

Augmentation Cystoplasty

Augmentation cystoplasty is used for resistant cases of bladder instability. In this major procedure, the bladder is opened up, and a strip of tissue that has been taken from the patient's intestine is placed as a patch over the opening to increase the volume capacity of the bladder.

❀ How Lilly Went Dancing Again ❀

Okay, now you know. I was 34 and leaking like a faucet. The first urologist I went to did some tests and recommended immediate surgery. My husband and I wanted to have another child, and I didn't want to commit to a C-section, so I sought a second opinion. That's when I met Dr. Bologna. He suggested we try a non-invasive approach first. It was a pessary, and it worked 100 percent of the time. After my second

continued on next page

{ Surgery and Other Options for Overactive Bladder,
Stress Urinary Incontinence, and Prolapse }

child, I elected to have the surgery, and it worked: I was dry for the first time since ... I don't remember when. To help keep me that way, he put me on The Sisterhood Plan. I'm 39 now and I'm still dry. With a daily commitment to pelvic floor exercises, I'm hoping I stay dry. Strike up the band.

CORRECTING STRESS URINARY INCONTINENCE

Of the three approaches to the treatment of stress urinary incontinence – pelvic floor therapy, fitting a *pessary*, and surgery – a well-fitting pessary can have the most immediate effect, followed closely by surgery.

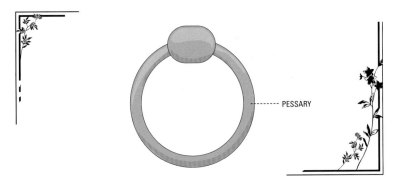

PESSARY

The Pessary – An Ancient Correction

References to the pessary in the literature appear early in 15th century Europe, but it may have an earlier Semitic origin. It came down to us as a small ring placed within the vagina to support prolapsed organs, but is also now used to control symptoms of stress urinary incontinence. Today, pessaries come in many shapes and styles and are made of plastic or silicone to support or correct the position of the bladder, urethra, uterus, or rectum. A health-care professional fits a patient for a pessary in the office.

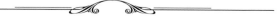

{ Prolapse And The Pelvic Floor }
A prolapse is a consequence of a weakened or damaged pelvic floor. As the pelvic floor muscles and ligaments holding the organs in place weaken, the bladder – or the uterus or the rectum – may begin to bulge down into the vagina (a vaginal prolapse) creating this hernia-like condition. Over time, if not treated, a prolapsed organ may descend into the vagina and literally turn the vagina inside out like a sock.

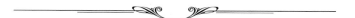

A pessary supports the pelvic floor to improve stress incontinence and reduces the bulge caused by one or more of the pelvic organs sagging through the pelvic floor (prolapse). It fits in the vagina just below the pubic bone, near the cervix, and has the following characteristics:

❀ A pessary's primary virtue is its simplicity – providing temporary or long-term relief without surgery.

❀ It doesn't work for everybody. Sometimes several types and sizes must be tried before one is found and works properly for the patient.

❀ It needs to come out periodically to be cleaned and re-inserted. Some patients can do this on their own; others will need to be seen by a nurse or other practitioner who will remove, clean, and re-insert it.

❀ It needs to be removed for sexual intercourse.

❀ You can't use a tampon while a pessary is in place.

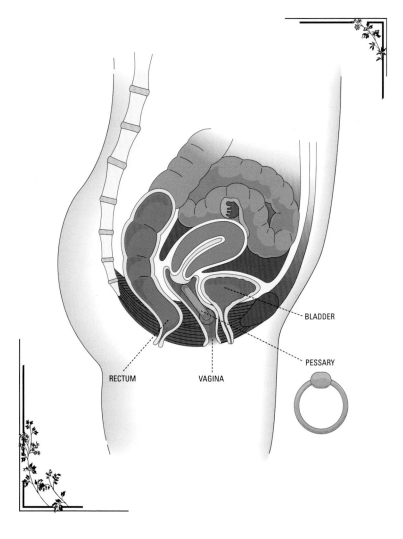

BLADDER

PESSARY

RECTUM

VAGINA

Surgical Correction of Stress Urinary Incontinence

The secret to surgical correction is to perform the right procedure for the right problem. Determining the right procedure to correct a problem starts with the initial discussion with the patient regarding the type of problem she is having – stress urinary incontinence, overactive bladder, or both? It's followed by the physical exam and bladder study to definitively identify the problem or problems.

The goal of all of the surgeries for stress urinary incontinence is to increase the tightness of the seal of the bladder neck and/or urethra when increased abdominal pressure is exerted on the bladder. In other words, to improve the seal the urethra makes when you cough, sneeze, run, or lift.

Retropubic Urethropexy
The Burch Procedure

The Burch procedure, developed by Dr. John C. Burch in 1958, has the most long-term follow-up data of any procedure for stress incontinence for patients with urethral hypermobility. The data reveal that more than 10 years after surgery, 80 to 93 percent of surgical patients are still dry. The Burch procedure supports the bladder neck and urethra by providing a backboard to support the urethra. This improves the urethra's ability to close when there is an increase in intra-abdominal pressure.

* The Burch procedure is performed through a low abdominal incision – the same incision used for a C-section or abdominal hysterectomy (a bikini-cut incision).

* It usually requires one or two days of a hospital admission.

* Because of the incision, most patients require at least two

weeks off from work.

❈ We ask patients to avoid heavy lifting, pulling, or pushing for at least eight weeks.

The Sling (or Hammock) Procedure

Like the Burch procedure, the Sling procedure has a long history and, as a surgical procedure, has benefited from significant advances in technique developed by a number of leading surgeons. The Sling procedure provides support underneath the urethra to increase the ability of the urethra to close.

Currently, there are two approaches to the procedure: the traditional Bladder-Neck Sling and the Mid-Urethral Sling.

The Bladder-Neck Sling

The traditional Bladder-Neck Sling remains the standard treatment for stress incontinence. It can be applied to all degrees of severity. The best candidates for this approach are those who may not respond to a Mid-Urethral Sling; those whose urethra closes very poorly (if at all), those who've had previous surgery that has failed or whose urethra was fixed in position.

The Mid-Urethral Sling

Introduced in 1996, the Mid-Urethral Sling delivers long-term outcomes comparable to the Burch procedure. But, for most patients, the most important feature of this approach is that it is done with smaller incisions and minimal recovery time.

The Mid-Urethral Sling supports the middle portion of a urethra that has a great deal of movement. It enables the urethra to stay closed despite increases in intra-abdominal pressure caused by a cough, sneeze, or lifting a heavy object.

Here is what you can expect if you elect the Mid-Urethral Sling and why it has become a preferred procedure:

- In the majority of cases, the procedure is done on an outpatient basis or with less than a 24-hour hospital stay, at most. Only minimal incisions of less than half an inch are required.

- Slings are made from a variety of materials, including medical-grade human- or animal-donated biologic material, your own tissue, or a polyester-like mesh that allows your own tissue to grow in and around it to become a part of you.

- The success rate for the Sling is high: up to 95 percent of patients are made dry or significantly improved. Long term, it has been shown that, in the majority of cases, if a patient is dry following the surgery, she will stay dry.

- The recovery period is four weeks, during which there can be no heavy lifting, pushing, or pulling. Patients will often return to work in a week, as long as they don't have to lift anything.

As with any surgery, there are certain concerns after sling surgery that include:

- Returning to normal voiding varies and may take longer for some patients.

- A small percentage of patients may have difficulty emptying their bladder completely after surgery and some require a second surgery to correct this problem.

- A small percentage of patients will not heal well over the synthetic mesh and require re-closure of the incision or removal of the mesh.

* Some patients who had overactive bladder symptoms before the operation find they worsen temporarily post-operatively.

* Some patients find that they develop new overactive bladder symptoms after surgery. This may often be the sign of incomplete bladder emptying or urinary tract infection.

* As with any surgery, there is a chance for complications. Patients are advised to review their progress with their health-care professionals. If a patient's incontinence continues, it may require a second surgery.

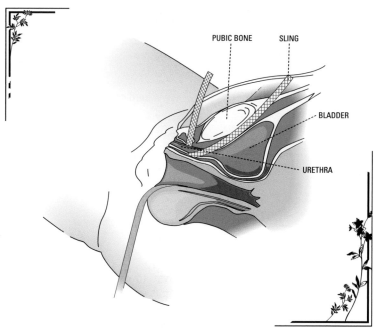

Sling Surgical Approaches

There are a number of excellent Slings available from various manufacturers. Their use commonly requires a small vaginal incision and two small, one-quarter-inch incisions made either above the pubic bone (the suprapubic approach) or outside the labial region (the transobturator approach).

The suprapubic approach passes a small needle from above the pubic bone underneath the urethra. The transobturator approach passes the needle through the obturator foramen, an opening in the pelvic bones between the labia and the thigh.

Here are the manufacturers and their products' names:

American Medical Systems	SPARC™ Monarc™ Bioarc™ MiniArc™	www.americanmedicalsystems.com
Bard	Uretex® Uretex® TO	www.bard.com
Boston Scientific	Lynx® Obtryx®	www.bostonscientific.com
Gynecare	TVT™ TVT-O™ TVT Secur™	www.gynecare.com
Coloplast Corporation	Aris™ T.O.T	www.us.coloplast.com

Urethral Bulking Injections

In addition to surgery, another way to correct stress urinary incontinence is to inject a material into the urethra around the sphincter. The injected material bulks up the urethra and augments its ability to make a tighter seal. The process is similar in nature to the practice of injecting material into one's facial lips for cosmetic purposes.

The ideal candidate for urethra injections is someone whose urethra is stable, that is, it doesn't move when pressure is exerted on the bladder as she coughs or sneezes. The problem here, known as *intrinsic sphincter deficiency*, is where the urethral sphincter simply isn't able to close completely.

Most patients will need two or three injections to improve their continence.

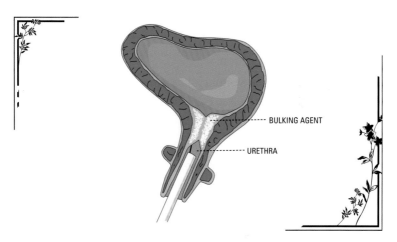

Three injectable implant materials are now commonly used:

* Contigen® – made from bovine (cow) collagen.

    ~ A skin test is required with this material to check for a possible allergic reaction.

    ~ Studies have shown a 65 percent improvement rate with Contigen.

    ~ Contigen's effectiveness decreases with time.

* Tegress™ – a new polymer bulking agent.

    ~ Injected as a liquid, Tegress becomes a spongy mass, providing increased closure ability.

    ~ The patient's body doesn't break down the Tegress material.

    ~ A long-term success rate has not yet been established.

❋ Coaptite® – biocompatible implant material.

   ~ Promotes tissue growth in urethra.

   ~ No skin test is required.

   ~ Two thirds of patients participating in a study done by the manufacturer reported improvement at 24 months.

Complications that might occur from the injections of these materials include:

❋ Urinary tract infection.

❋ Discomfort when voiding.

❋ Short-term difficulty voiding.

Artificial Urinary Sphincter

The artificial urinary sphincter (AUS), most commonly used in male incontinence, is reserved for the most difficult cases of stress urinary incontinence. Produced by American Medical Systems, the AUS is designed to place a cuff around the urethra. This cuff gently squeezes the urethra closed, which acts like the patient's sphincter. It stays closed until a patient needs to urinate. She would then pump a small device (about the size of an almond) located in the area of her labia. This allows the sphincter cuff to open. The patient has approximately three minutes to empty her bladder as the cuff slowly re-closes. The AUS has a very high success rate and has been used for 35 years.

CORRECTING PROLAPSE

There are three approaches to the problem of a prolapse: watchful waiting, fitting a pessary, and surgery.

❋ How the Way Was Cleared for Anna ❋

I made an appointment to see Dr. Bologna. He gave me a couple of options to consider in dealing with the bladder prolapse: wear a pessary to support the bladder from within the vagina, or undergo surgery to re-support the bladder in place. The thing about the pessary, aside from the fact that it seemed to work pretty well for me, is that I had to take it out for intercourse. And, frankly, I didn't want the bother, so I went for the surgery – but not at first. While I was making up my mind, Dr. Bologna suggested that I give pelvic floor muscle therapy a try. It involved more than just Kegels. I went along with it, and I wished I had known about it sooner. But I made up my mind to have the surgery, anyway. The operation required attaching the bladder and vagina to the deep ligaments in my pelvis and adding a mesh sling under my bladder for support. I was in and out of the hospital in less than 24 hours. I'm really relieved. The way had been cleared for my husband and me to resume our golf and traveling. I've continued the pelvic muscle exercises, and the intimacy we'd shared for more than 40 years is feeling like it used to in earlier days.

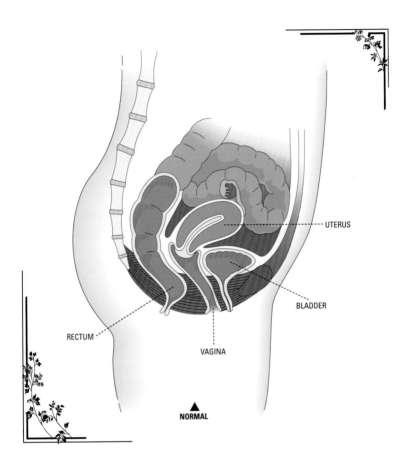

UTERUS

BLADDER

RECTUM

VAGINA

▲
NORMAL

When a prolapse requires surgical correction, it's important to identify all areas of weakness in the pelvic floor and fix them all. The operation can be approached through the abdomen or the vagina.

The abdominal approach has long been considered the gold standard. Using mesh to reinforce the pelvic floor, it offers good support and a low failure rate. Its only disadvantage is the

{ Surgery and Other Options for Overactive Bladder,
Stress Urinary Incontinence, and Prolapse }

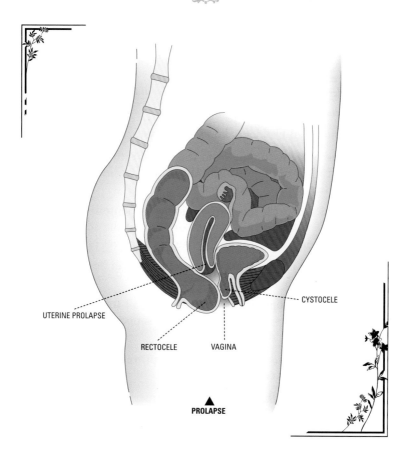

UTERINE PROLAPSE

CYSTOCELE

RECTOCELE   VAGINA

▲
PROLAPSE

abdominal incision, which some women understandably would choose to avoid if possible. However, patients frequently require a combination of both abdominal and vaginal surgery.

Newer, effective vaginal approaches, which also apply mesh to reinforce support, are now available. A laproscopic approach is also used.

the
ACCIDENTAL SISTERHOOD

Surgical correction of prolapse deals directly with what can fall down and what can be done to re-support it:

Bladder Prolapse – Loss of support on the anterior side (front wall) of the vagina.

- A prolapsed bladder is known as a cystocele.
- If the bulge is coming from the top of the vagina, it can be due to loss of support from the middle or sides of the ligament support structures.
- When support is lost in the middle, a traditional anterior repair can be performed with or without the addition of mesh along with a Sling Procedure to correct incontinence.
- If support is lost on the sides, the repair can be performed through a vaginal or abdominal incision.
- Rebuilding support involves repairing a patient's own support tissues and, at times, adding support with the use of a synthetic or biologic mesh.
- New procedures are available to improve outcomes and decrease recovery time.
- Avaulta™ by C.R. Bard, Perigee® by American Medical Systems (AMS), and Prolift® by Johnson & Johnson provide an all-vaginal approach to re-supporting the bladder and vagina using the deep ligaments in the pelvis and adding mesh for further support. It requires a hospital stay of less than 24 hours.

Enterocele – Loss of support at the apex of the vagina.

An enterocele is a loss of support at the apex (or top) of the vagina. A hernia appears at this point, allowing the bowel to push into the vagina. An enterocele can happen with or without a uterus in place. An enterocele can be corrected via an abdominal or vaginal approach. At the time of an enterocele repair, it's often necessary for the patient to require correction of a vaginal prolapse.

Uterine Prolapse / Vaginal Prolapse — Loss of support for the uterus.
Uterine and vaginal prolapses result from a stretching or a weakening of the ligaments that hold the uterus in place. Vaginal prolapse takes place after a woman has had a hysterectomy (removal of the uterus).

A number of questions must be considered when a patient with uterine prolapse consults her health-care professional.
- Does the patient have a medical reason requiring removal of the uterus?
  - ~ Abnormal uterine bleeding?
  - ~ Uterine or cervical cancer or pre-cancerous cells?
- Has the patient had a recent screening evaluation for potential uterine or cervical cancer?

Differing options exist regarding removal of the uterus at the time of prolapse correction. Essentially, the same surgeries can be done with the uterus in place or removed. We do know that if a patient is having a hysterectomy and she has uterine prolapse, something should be done at the time of the procedure to re-support the top of the vagina.

Surgical correction of uterine and vaginal prolapse is done at the top of the vagina, which can be re-supported by an abdominal or vaginal approach. There are several surgical approaches.

The abdominal approach can be done with the uterus in place (*abdominal sacral hysteropexy*) or without the uterus in place (*abdominal sacral colpopexy*).

❋ These procedures are done through an abdominal incision at the time of a hysterectomy for uterine prolapse, or as a separate procedure if the patient has already had a hysterectomy. It involves the placement of a soft synthetic or biologic mesh material at the top of the vagina and connecting it to the area at the base of the spine above the tailbone. Every effort should be made to understand a patient's urethral function to correct or prevent stress urinary incontinence.

Sacrospinous ligament fixation/Uterosacral ligament fixation/Iliococygeal ligament suspension.

❋ These are vaginal procedures that can be used to correct vaginal or uterine prolapse. They are done by attaching the top of the vagina or cervix to ligaments deep in the pelvis to provide support. In some cases with the attachment, a woman may experience lower back pain or pain during intercourse.

❋ Mesh systems, such as Apogee® by AMS, may also be used to correct uterine or vaginal prolapse.

Posterior vaginal wall prolapse (rectocele).

❋ When the support tissues on the bottom (or posterior) side of the vagina have loosened, it allows the rectum to bulge into the vagina. This form of prolapse is known as rectocele.

❋ Women with this problem typically complain about needing to "splint" – that is, having to put a finger in their vaginas to push their rectums back into place in order to have a bowel movement. They will also resort to rocking forward or pushing in the perineum to relieve themselves.

❀ Rectocele repairs are done through a vaginal approach. Surgery involves repairing the support tissue. Sometimes mesh is used to help increase that support. If it's associated with a loss of vaginal support, the Apogee, Avaulta, and Prolift systems can be used to support the top of the vagina and provide mesh to supplement the repair. At the time of repair of the bottom side of the vagina, the perineal body is also re-supported.

What to expect after pelvic floor surgery.

The most common complaints expressed after the types of pelvic floor surgeries just described include:

❀ Constipation – This is a constant battle because of the location of the surgery, the decrease in physical activity, and the use of pain medication. We encourage patients to increase their fluid intake and use a stool softener every day. Occasionally, we prescribe medicines to help or we recommend a high-fiber diet. (See **Healthy Bowel Function** and **Fiber Facts** in the **Appendix**.)

❀ Urinary urgency – As we mentioned, any pelvic surgery can increase urgency for a period of time.

❀ Vaginal spotting – It's very common for patients to spot for two to four weeks after surgery.

As with the use of any synthetic mesh, a small percentage of patients will not heal well over the mesh and will require re-closure of the incision or removal of the mesh. We will routinely start patients on vaginal estrogens – typically, one month prior to surgery – to help improve healing and decrease discomfort with intercourse. Intercourse may be uncomfortable for a period of time, and most health-care professionals ask patients to wait eight to 12 weeks after vaginal surgery.

There shouldn't be any discomfort after three months, but if it persists – don't be shy – your health-care professional *needs* to know because it can be a symptom of mesh exposure or an infection.

POSTSCRIPT TO SURGERY AND STAYING DRY FOR GOOD

Surgical corrections for incontinence and prolapse are constantly evolving. New techniques and procedures are providing improved outcomes and shorter recovery times. The goal is to make every patient dry and to correct every prolapse. Although a small percentage of patients require repeat procedures, this can be reduced even further with the addition of pelvic floor therapy.

Unlike orthopedic procedures, where patients expect to go through post-surgery physical therapy, patients who have had pelvic floor surgery often believe that nothing more is required of them. They're eager to get on with their lives, and that's understandable. But they can significantly improve their post-surgery recovery if they also undergo physical therapy of their pelvic floor.

As surgical techniques improve, we are improving patient outcomes by encouraging patients to strengthen their pelvic floor muscles both pre- and post-surgery. The Sisterhood Plan is a new and unique approach to pelvic floor therapy that will not only get better results sooner, but will also encourage lifelong compliance with a manageable and patient-friendly regimen.

{ Surgery and Other Options for Overactive Bladder, Stress Urinary Incontinence, And Prolapse }

Don't stop here, though. Continue your commitment by visiting our Web site, *www.AccidentalSisterhood.com*, where you'll find up-to-date information on new surgical and non-surgical options for pelvic floor health – and a host of other issues important to this vital subject. To find out more about us, log on today.

As we've said, *The Accidental Sisterhood* is a response to an enormous problem facing many women – a problem that is too often ignored and vastly underestimated. We believe that every woman can benefit from The Sisterhood Plan . . . that you can benefit from it.

But even more than that, this book presents the full array of options available to you to make you dry and keep you that way. Healing and strengthening your pelvic floor – everything about it, not just the symptoms of urgency or incontinence – is what we set out to do. Our goal is to help you regain control of a fundamental part of your body – your pelvic floor. If we've encouraged you to undertake The Sisterhood Plan, or to seek medical care for your problem, then it's by no accident that we've succeeded.

Share your success with us, and help us tell all those other enduring women who belong to The Accidental Sisterhood that they're not alone.

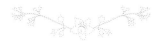

the
ACCIDENTAL SISTERHOOD

{ Appendix }

Bladder Irritating Medications . . . Healthy Bowel Function . . . Fiber Facts . . .
Caffeine Content In Consumer Beverages, O-T-C Medicines, and Desserts

BLADDER IRRITATING MEDICATIONS[8]

Diuretics (water pills) *Examples:* Esidrix® (hydrochlorothiaxide-HCTZ) Lasix® (furosemide) Maxide® (HCTZ-triamterene)	**Effects:** More urine produced, frequency, urgency.

Sedatives, muscle relaxants *Examples:* Valium® (diazepam) Librium® (chlordiazepoxide) Atvian® (lorazepam)	**Effects:** More urine produced, frequency, urgency.

---

[8] Adapted from "Classes of Drugs Which May Contribute to Incontinence," *Your Personal Guide to Bladder Health*, published by the National Association for Continence, 2001.

Narcotics *Examples:* Percoset® (oxycodone-AAP) Demerol®	**Effects:** Sedation, drowsiness, bladder relaxes retaining urine, difficulty in starting the urinary stream, straining to urinate, voiding with a weak stream, frequency.

Antihistamines *Examples:* Benadryl® (diphenhydramine) **Anticholinergics** *Examples:* Pro-Banthine® (propantheline) **Antipsychotics/Antidepressants** *Examples:* Elavil® (amitriptyline) Prolixin® (fluphenazine) Haldol® (haloperidol) Prozac® (fluoxetine HCL) **Calcium channelblockers** *Examples:* Calan® (verapamil) Procardia® (nifedipine) Cardizem® (diltiazem)	**Effects:** Retention of urine because bladder relaxes; sometimes more urine produced, difficulty in starting the stream, straining to urinate, voiding a weak stream, leaking.

Alpha adrenergic agonist *Examples:* Entex®, Sudafed® (pseudoephedrine) Dexatrim® (phenylpropanolomine)	**Effects:** Increases the resistance of the bladder outlet muscle, urinary retention, frequency, weak stream, leaking.

Alpha adrenergic antagonist *Examples:* Hytrin® (terazosin) Cardura® (doxazosin)	**Effects:** Relaxes the bladder sphincter muscle, leaking when coughing, sneezing, laughing, etc.

Over-the-counter cold remedies *Examples:* Nyquil®, Theraflu®, Alka Seltzer Plus Cold Relief®, Afrin® nose drops	**Effects:** Depending on the medication: bladder muscle contracts or relaxes, causing urinary retention or leaking.

HEALTHY BOWEL FUNCTION

After you eat, it takes from one to four days for the food to travel through your entire digestive system. The waste products (stool) are propelled by intestinal contractions from the small intestine to the large intestine and then into the rectum, where the stool is stored until you have a bowel movement. The rectum stretches and expands as it fills, but doesn't release the stool until the appropriate time because of two muscles that act like drawstrings, the external and internal anal sphincters. We have voluntary control of the external but not the internal anal sphincter. When you are conscious of the urge to have a bowel movement, you sit on the toilet, relax the muscles of your pelvic floor and the external anal sphincter, and push without straining. Evacuation of the bowel then takes place.

Stool Consistency

Diet plays a large part in determining the consistency of your stool. A diet rich in fiber is ideal. (See **Fiber Facts** in the **Appendix** for a list of foods and their fiber content.)

Stool can be loose and runny, soft and moderately bulky, or hard. *Soft and moderately bulky stool is the easiest to eliminate.* If your stool is loose and runny it is harder to keep it in the rectum without leakage. In this respect, it is like gas, which your body expels all day long. Strengthening your pelvic floor muscles will help improve your ability to keep the anus tightly closed to prevent leakage of stool. If your stool is too hard, it is harmful to the pelvic floor muscles as you strain to push the stool out of the rectum.

Ideally, you want your stool to be "fluffy floaters" – that is, a stool that floats in the toilet and does not sink and "hide."

It's important to identify problem foods. You may wish to eliminate the problem foods from your diet. Some foods that can be irritating to the bowel include:

- ❀ Lactose (found in many dairy products)
- ❀ Chocolate
- ❀ Greasy or fatty foods
- ❀ Foods containing sorbitol (sweetener found in some breath mints, gum, or sugar-free candy can have a laxative effect)
- ❀ Spicy foods

It's also important to eat nutritious meals at regular, scheduled times.

Loose Stools

Loose stools, or diarrhea, can be a symptom of gastrointestinal diseases. It usually clears up after a few days.

When it doesn't it may be more serious, and you should see your health-care professional. There are a number of over-the-counter remedies for loose stools, and they work reasonably well. But it's best not to become dependent on them. Instead, there are a variety of dietary modifications, such as eating certain foods that can thicken your stool:

- Foods containing pectin (bananas, applesauce, and marshmallows)

- Starchy foods (rice, bread, potatoes)

- Cheese

- Peanut butter

- Fiber additives (Metamucil®, Citrucel®, Per Diem Fiber®, Unifiber®, Benefiber®, and Konsyl®) help by attracting and absorbing fluid in the intestines. The usual dose for adults is one to two teaspoons dissolved in water, one to three times a day. If you use a fiber supplement, be sure to read the directions on the package and take with plenty of water. Fiber supplements are not recommended for children under six years of age. It has been reported that psyllium, the major ingredient of Metamucil, can absorb certain medications, decreasing their effectiveness. It is best not to take psyllium within two hours of taking other medications, particularly digoxin (Cardoxin®, Digitek®), warfarin (Coumadin®), and salicylates, such as aspirin.

A diet rich in high-fiber foods is necessary for people who routinely have loose stools, as well as those with constipation. For those with loose stools, natural fiber in foods absorbs water and swells, thus bulking up the stool and making it more solid.

In constipation, the situation is somewhat reversed: there is too little water in the stool, causing the stool to become more compacted and hard. Adding more fiber and fluids to the diet tends to draw water into the bowel, thus softening and bulking up the stool, which makes it easier to eliminate. Adults should have 20 to 30 grams of fiber in their daily diets.

Be aware that as you begin to increase the amount of fiber in your diet you may experience an increase in gas and bloating. This condition will lessen in time, so be patient and, perhaps, increase the addition of fiber more slowly.

Hard Stools/Constipation
To soften the stool, gradually increase the amount of high-fiber foods you eat each day. Below are some foods that are high in fiber content:

- High-fiber cereals (Fiber One®, All-Bran®, Raisin Bran®, Kashi Go Lean Crunch®)

- Fruits and vegetables

- Nuts

- Bran formula: one cup of unprocessed miller's bran + one cup of applesauce + one-fourth cup of prune juice. Begin with one to two tablespoons per day of the bran formula and increase daily dose by one tablespoon each week until regular evacuation of soft-formed stool is established. Drink eight ounces of fluid immediately after fiber consumption.

- Fiber additives (Metamucil, Citrucel, Per Diem Fiber, Unifiber, Benefiber, and Konsyl) will help soften your stool. These substances work by attracting and absorbing fluid. The usual dose is one to two teaspoons dissolved in water, one to three times a day. If you use a fiber supplement, be sure to read the directions on the package and take with plenty of water.

❋ Adequate fluid intake. We recommend drinking eight eight-ounce glasses of fluid, including water and other non-irritating fluids, every day. This is especially important as you increase your fiber intake.

❋ Physical exercise, such as walking or riding a bicycle, will stimulate intestinal contractions.

❋ Respond promptly to the urge to have a bowel movement, since this is when the stool is easiest to eliminate.

❋ Establish a normal schedule. Attempt to have a bowel movement at the same time each day. The time should be soon after a meal to take advantage of normal digestive contractions caused by eating. After breakfast is often best, but choose a time based on your previous habits.

❋ Do not sit on the toilet for more than 10 to 15 minutes. If you are unsuccessful, go do something else and try again later. Remember that physical activity stimulates your bowel.

❋ The height of the toilet and your position can affect the ease or difficulty you experience while attempting to have a bowel movement. Try putting a small step stool under your feet or leaning forward. Avoid tall toilets whenever possible.

❋ It may be necessary to strain or bear down a little to start your bowel moving, but *do not* hold your breath. If you are used to straining and have been doing so for a long time, this may be a difficult habit to unlearn, but it's very important. Continued straining is harmful to the pelvic floor muscles and may actually worsen the problem. Without realizing it, you may also be tightening the muscles instead of relaxing them, as you need to. Learning to relax the muscles at the appropriate time may be part of a physical therapy treatment that you may elect to pursue.

Keep in mind that the level of emotional stress and anxiety you experience affects your bowel. Constipation commonly occurs from chronic stress or nervousness. However, it's common to have loose stools during bouts of high stress as well. All of us experience periods of stress and anxiety, but every person who is affected by it responds individually. Keeping your stress levels to a minimum and learning how to manage your stress is important in maintaining healthy bowel habits.

FIBER FACTS

Adding fiber to your diet is easy. Here are some tips that can help you get started:

- Substitute high-fiber foods (whole grains, brown rice, fruits, and vegetables, especially fresh fruits and vegetables that are eaten raw with the skin) instead of low-fiber foods (white bread, white rice, candy, and chips).
- Eat high-fiber foods at every meal. For example, bran flakes topped with sliced fruit and low-fat milk is a great, high-fiber way to start your day.
- Add fiber to your diet slowly.
- Drink plenty of water while consuming a high-fiber diet to prevent constipation. If you are still falling short of your fiber goal of 20 to 30 grams per day, consider adding a fiber supplement.

FOODS	SERVING SIZE	FIBER GRAMS per serving	CALORIES per serving
Breads			
Whole wheat	1 slice	2.11	70
White	1 slice	0.50	70
Rye	1 slice	1.72	70
Cereal			
Oat bran	1 ounce	4.06	110
Shredded wheat	1 ounce	2.64	90
Corn flakes	1 ounce	0.45	110
Rice			
Brown	1/2 cup	5.27	109
White	1/2 cup	1.42	133
Spaghetti (uncooked)	2 ounces	2.56	220
Vegetables (cooked, unless otherwise noted)			
Broccoli	1/2 cup	2.58	22
Brussels sprouts	1/2 cup	2.00	30
Corn	1/2 cup	3.03	89
Eggplant	1/2 cup	0.96	13
Green peas	1/2 cup	3.36	67
Lettuce (raw)	1/2 cup	0.24	5
Potato (baked w/skin)	1/2 cup	2.97	57
Spinach	1/2 cup	2.07	21
Squash (baked)	1/2 cup	2.87	57
Tomato (raw)	1/2 cup	1.17	19
Zucchini	1/2 cup	1.26	14
Beans			
Green (canned)	1/2 cup	1.89	20
Kidney	1/2 cup	5.48	100
Lima	1/2 cup	4.25	90
Pinto	1/2 cup	5.93	101

cont. on next page

FOODS	SERVING SIZE	FIBER GRAMS per serving	CALORIES per serving
Fresh fruits			
Apple (w/peel)	1 medium	2.76	81
Apricots	1 cup	3.13	74
Banana	1 medium	2.19	105
Blackberries	1 cup	7.20	74
Boysenberries	1 cup	7.20	74
Grapefruit	1 medium	3.61	92
Grapes	1 cup	1.12	114
Orange	1 medium	3.14	65
Pear (w/peel)	1 medium	4.32	98
Prunes (canned)	1 cup	13.76	246
Raspberries	1 cup	7.50	62
Strawberries	1 cup	3.87	46
Watermelon	1 slice	1.93	152

CAFFEINE CONTENT IN CONSUMER BEVERAGES, O-T-C MEDICINES, AND DESSERTS

Caffeine is similar in structure to adenosine, a chemical found in the brain that slows its activity. Since the two chemicals compete, the more caffeine you drink, the less adenosine is available. That's why caffeine temporarily heightens concentration and wards off fatigue.

Within 30 to 60 minutes of drinking a cup of coffee, caffeine reaches peak concentrations in the bloodstream. It typically takes four to six hours for its effects to wear off.

Smokers remove caffeine from their blood twice as fast as

nonsmokers. That may be why smokers tend to drink more coffee.

The average American adult consumes about 200 milligrams (mg) of caffeine a day, and the top 10 percent consume an average of 400 mg, according to The Coca-Cola Company in Atlanta.

As little as 200 mg of caffeine is enough to make some people feel nervous and anxious. It might take even less for cola-guzzling kids.

The typical American drinks about two cups of coffee a day. In 1962, when coffee consumption hit its peak, three cups was typical. With the advent of Starbucks and other gourmet coffee shops, consumption among younger adults is again probably reaching levels of the peak-consumption period.

Coffee accounts for about 75 percent of the caffeine we consume. Tea makes up about 15 percent, soft drinks about 10 percent, and chocolate about two percent.

COFFEE

Starbucks Coffee, grande (16 oz.)	550 mg
Starbucks Coffee, tall (12 oz.)	375 mg
Starbucks Coffee, short (8 oz.)	250 mg
Starbucks Caffe Americano, short (8 oz.)	350 mg
Starbucks Caffe Latte, short (8 oz.) or tall (12 oz.)	350 mg
Starbucks Caffe Mocha, short (8 oz.) or tall (12 oz.)	350 mg
Starbucks Espresso, double (2 oz.)	700 mg
Starbucks Coffee, decaf, grande (16 oz.)	10 mg

cont. on next page

the
ACCIDENTAL SISTERHOOD

cont. from previous page

COFFEE

Coffee, non-gourmet (8 oz.) . . . . .135 mg

Coffee, decaf, non-gourmet (8 oz.) . . . . .5 mg

Coffee, instant (8 oz.) . . . . .95 mg

General Foods International Coffee, Cafe Vienna (8 oz.) . . . . .90 mg

Maxwell House Cappuccino, Mocha (8 oz.) . . . . .60-65 mg

General Foods International Coffee, Swiss Mocha (8 oz.) . . . . . . .55 mg

Maxwell House Cappuccino, French Vanilla
or Irish Cream (8 oz.) . . . . .45-50 mg

Maxwell House Cappuccino, Amaretto (8 oz.) . . . . .25-30 mg

General Foods International Coffee,
Viennese Chocolate Café (8 oz.) . . . . .26 mg

Maxwell House Cappuccino, decaffeinated (8 oz.) . . . . .3-6 mg

TEAS

Celestial Seasonings Iced Lemon Ginseng Tea (16-oz. Bottle) . . .100 mg

Bigelow Raspberry Royale Tea (8 oz.) . . . . .83 mg

Tea, leaf or bag (8 oz.) . . . . .50 mg

Snapple Iced Tea, all varieties (16-oz. Bottle) . . . . .48 mg

Lipton Natural Brew Iced Tea Mix, unsweetened (8 oz.) . . . . . .25-45 mg

Lipton Tea (8 oz.) . . . . .35-40 mg

Lipton Iced Tea, assorted varieties (16-oz. bottle) . . . . .18-40 mg

Lipton Natural Brew Iced Tea Mix, sweetened (8 oz.) . . . . .15-35 mg

Nestea Pure Sweetened Iced Tea (16-oz. bottle) . . . . .34 mg

Tea, green (8 oz.) . . . . .30 mg

cont. on next page

{ Appendix }

cont. from previous page

TEAS

Arizona Iced Tea, assorted varieties (16-oz. bottle)	15-30 mg
Lipton Soothing Moments Blackberry Tea (8 oz.)	25 mg
Nestea Pure Lemon Sweetened Iced Tea (16-oz. bottle)	22 mg
Tea, instant (8 oz.)	15 mg
Lipton Natural Brew Iced Tea Mix, diet (8 oz.)	10-15 mg
Lipton Natural Brew Iced Tea Mix, decaffeinated (8 oz.)	5 mg
Celestial Seasonings Herbal Tea, all varieties (8 oz.)	0 mg
Celestial Seasonings Herbal Iced Tea, bottled (16-oz. bottle)	0 mg
Lipton Soothing Moments Peppermint Tea (8 oz.)	0 mg

SOFT DRINKS

Red Bull (8 oz.)	80 mg
Josta (12 oz.)	58 mg
Mountain Dew (12 oz.)	55 mg
Surge (12 oz.)	51 mg
Diet Coke (12 oz.)	47 mg
Coca-Cola (12 oz.)	45 mg
Dr. Pepper, regular or diet (12 oz.)	41 mg
Sunkist Orange Soda (12 oz.)	40 mg
Pepsi-Cola (12 oz.)	37 mg
Barq's Root Beer (12 oz.)	23 mg
7-UP or Diet 7-UP (12 oz.)	0 mg
Barq's Diet Root Beer (12 oz.)	0 mg
Caffeine-free Coca-Cola or Diet Coke (12 oz.)	0 mg

cont. on next page

the
ACCIDENTAL SISTERHOOD

SOFT DRINKS

Caffeine-free Pepsi or Diet Pepsi (12 oz.) ....0 mg

Minute Maid Orange Soda (12 oz.) ....0 mg

Mug Root Beer (12 oz.) ....0 mg

Sprite or Diet Sprite (12 oz.) ....0 mg

CAFFEINATED WATERS

Java Water (16.9 oz.) ....125 mg

Krank 20 (16.9 oz.) ....100 mg

Aqua Blast (16.9 oz.) ....90 mg

Water Joe (16.9 oz.) ....60-70 mg

Aqua Java (16.9 oz.) ....50-60 mg

OTC DRUGS

NoDoz, maximum strength, or Vivarin 1 tablet ....200 mg

Excedrin, 2 tablets ....130 mg

NoDoz, regular strength 1 tablet ....100 mg

Anacin, 2 tablets ....64 mg

FROZEN DESSERTS

Ben & Jerry's No-Fat Coffee Fudge Frozen Yogurt (1 cup) .... 85 mg

Starbucks Coffee Ice Cream, assorted flavors (1 cup) ....40-60 mg

cont. on next page

cont. from previous page

FROZEN DESSERTS

Häagen-Dazs Coffee Ice Cream (1 cup) . . . . .58 mg

Häagen-Dazs Coffee Frozen Yogurt, fat-free (1 cup) . . . . .40 mg

Häagen-Dazs Coffee Fudge Ice Cream, low-fat (1 cup) . . . . .30 mg

Starbucks Frappuccino Bar (1 bar, 2.5 oz.) .15 mg

Healthy Choice Cappuccino Chocolate Chunk
or Cappuccino Mocha Fudge Ice Cream (1 cup) . . . . .8 mg

YOGURTS, ONE CONTAINER

Dannon Coffee Yogurt (8 oz.) . . . . .45 mg

Yoplait Cafe Au Lait Yogurt (6 oz.) . . . . .5 mg

Dannon Light Cappuccino Yogurt (8 oz.) . . . . .1 mg

Stonyfield Farm Cappuccino Yogurt (8 oz.) .0 mg

CHOCOLATES

Hershey's Special Dark Chocolate Bar (1 bar, 1.5 oz.) . . . . .31 mg

Perugina Milk Chocolate Bar
with Cappuccino Filling (1/3 bar, 1.2 oz.) . . . . .24 mg

Hershey's Bar (milk chocolate) (1 bar, 1.5 oz.) . . . . .10 mg

Coffee Nips (hard candy - 2 pieces) . . . . .6 mg

Cocoa or Hot Chocolate (8 oz.) . . . . .5 mg

Chocolate, dark, bittersweet, semi-sweet (1 oz.) . . . . .20 mg

Sources: Center for Science in the Public Interest, National Coffee Association, National Soft Drink Association, Tea Council of the USA, and information provided by food, beverage, and pharmaceutical companies, and H.R. Roberts (1996) "Caffeine Consumption." Food Chemistry and Toxicology, vol. 34, pp. 119-129.

{ Further Reading and Reference }

Incontinence and Bladder Control

Female Urology, Urogynecology, and Voiding Dysfunction, S. P. Vasavanda, M.D., et. al. Marcel Dekker, New York, 2005

The Incontinence Solution: Answers for Women of All Ages, W. H. Parker, et. al. Fireside, New York, 2002

Mayo Clinic on Managing Incontinence, P. Pettit, editor. Mayo Clinic, Rochester, NY, 2005

Overcoming Bladder Disorders, R. Chalker and K.E. Whitmore, M.D. Harper Perennial, New York, 1991

Overcoming Overactive Bladder: Your Complete Self-Care Guide,
D. K. Newman and A. J. Wein, M.D. New Harbinger
Publications, Oakland, CA, 2004

*Conquering Incontinence: A New and Physical Approach
to a Freer Lifestyle*, P. Dornan. Allen & Unwin, 2003

*I Laughed So Hard I Peed My Pants: A Woman's Essential
Guide for Improved Bladder Control*, K. Berzuk. IPPC, 2002

Women's Waterworks: Curing Incontinence, P. Chiarelli.
George Perry, 2002

Your Personal Guide to Bladder Health, National Association
for Continence, 2001

7 Steps to Normal Bladder Control, E. Vierck. Harbor Press,
Inc., Gig Harbor, WA, 1998

Pelvic Floor Fitness and Health

The Female Pelvis: Anatomy & Exercises, B. Calais-Germain.
Eastland Press, Seattle, 2003

The V Book: A Doctor's Guide to Complete Vulvovaginal Health,
Elizabeth Gunther Stewart, M.D., and Paula Spencer. Bantam
Books, New York, 2002

Vaginas: An Owner's Manual, Carol Livoti, M.D., and Elizabeth
Topp. Thunder's Mouth Press, New York, 2004

Saving the Whole Woman: Natural Alternatives to Surgery for Pelvic Organ Prolapse and Urinary Incontinence, A. K. Kent. Bridgeworks, Albuquerque, NM, 2003

Pelvic Floor Re-education: Principles and Practice, B. Schüssler, et. al. Springer-Verlag, London, 1994

Pelvic Power for Men and Women: Mind/Body Exercises for Strength, Flexibility, Posture, and Balance, Eric Franklin. Princeton Book Company, Publishers, Hightstown, NJ, 2003

Fitness for the Pelvic Floor, Beate Carrière, PT. Thieme, New York, 2002

Beyond Kegels, Second Edition, J. A. Hulme. Phoenix Publishing Company, Missoula, MT, 2002

Ever Since I Had My Baby, R. Goldberg. Three Rivers Press, New York, 2003

Pelvic Health & Childbirth: What Every Woman Needs to Know, M. Murphy, M.D., and C. L. Wasson. Prometheus Books, Amherst, NY, 2003

Sexuality

For Women Only: A Revolutionary Guide to Reclaiming Your Sex Life, J. Berman, M.D., and L. Berman, Ph.D. Henry Holt, New York, 2001

Human Sexual Response, W. H. Masters and V. E. Johnson. Little, Brown, Boston, 1966

Secrets of the Sexually Satisfied Woman: Ten Keys to Unlocking Ultimate Pleasure, L. Berman, Ph.D., and J. Berman, M.D., Hyperion, New York, 2005

Sexual Behavior in the Human Female, Kinsey, A.C., et al. Indiana University Press, Bloomington, Reprint Edition, 1998.

Male and Female Sexual Dysfunction, A. D. Seftel, M.D., editor. Mosby, New York, 2004

General Reference

Atlas of Human Anatomy, Frank H. Netter, M.D. CIBA-GEIGY Corporation, West Caldwell, NJ, 1989

{ ONLINE RESOURCES }

Online Health and Lifestyle Information

InContiNet
www.incontinet.com

Institute of Medicine of the National Academies
www.iom.edu

iVillage (Women's Health and Well-Being)
www.ivillage.com

Medline Plus®
U.S. National Library of Medicine
National Institutes of Health
www.nlm.nih.gov/medlineplus

National Association for Continence
www.nafc.org

National Institutes of Health
www.health.nih.gov

National Institute on Aging, NIH
www.nia.nih.gov

National Kidney and Urologic Disease Information
www.kidney.niddk.nih.gov

National Women's Health Resource Center
www.healthywomen.org

RealAge
www.realage.com

The Simon Foundation for Continence
www.simonfoundation.org

The Whole Woman (prolapse information)
www.wholewoman.com

WebMD
www.webmd.com

Women's Sexual Wellness
Association of Reproductive Health Professionals and
National Women's Health Resource Center
www.nurtureyournature.org

Online Product Sources
Good Vibrations (sex education and erotica)
www.goodvibes.com

Medical Organizations
American Academy of Family Physicians
www.familydoctor.org

American College of Obstetricians and Gynecologists
www.acog.org

American Medical Women's Association
www.amwa–doc.org

American Physical Therapy Association
www.apta.org

American Urogynecologic Society (AUGS)
www.augs.org

American Urological Association (AUA)
www.urologyhealth.org
www.auanet.org

AUA Foundation, Inc.
www.afud.org

Herman & Wallace, Inc.
Pelvic Rehabilitation Institute
www.pelvicrehab.com

International Continence Society (ICS)
www.continet.org

Society for Urodynamics & Female Urology
www.sufuorg.com

Pharmaceuticals

Ditropan® XL (oxybutynin chloride)
Ortho-McNeil Pharmaceutical, Inc.
www.ditropan.com

Detrol® LA(tolterodine tartrate)
Pfizer, Inc.
www.bladderinfo.com
www.detrolla.com

Enablex® (darifenacin)
Novartis
www.enablex.com

Oxytrol® (oxybutynin transdermal system)
Watson Pharma, Inc.
www.bladdercontrol.com
www.oxytrol.com

SANCTURA® (trospium chloride)
Esprit Pharmaceuticals, Inc.
Indevus Pharmaceuticals, Inc.
www.sanctura.com

VESIcare® (solifenacin succinate)
Astellas Pharma Inc.
The GlaxoSmithKline Group of Companies
www.vesicare.com

Estrace® (estradiol vaginal cream)
Warner Chilcott PLC
www.estrace.com

Premarin® (conjugated estrogens – hormonal vaginal cream)
Wyeth Pharmaceuticals, Inc.
www.premarin.com

Vagifem® (estradiol vaginal tablets)
Novo Nordisk Inc.
www.vagifem.com

Medical Devices

SPARC™, Monarc™, BioArc™, MiniArc™ (Surgical Slings)
Perigee®, Apogee® (Prolapse Repair)
AUS (Artificial Urinary Sphincter)
American Medical System (AMS)
www.americanmedicalsystems.com

Lynx®, Obtryx® (Surgical Slings)
Coaptite® (Injectable Bulking Agent)
Boston Scientific
www.bostonscientific.com

Uretex® Uretex®TO (Surgical Slings)
Avaulta™ (Prolapse Repair)
Contigen®, Tegress® (Injectable Bulking Agents)
C. R. Bard, Inc.
www.bard.com

Gynecare TVT™, TVT-O™, TVT Secur™ (Surgical Slings)
Prolift (Prolapse Repair)
Ethicon, Inc. (Johnson & Johnson)
www.gynecare.com

Aris™ T.O.T. (Surgical Sling)
Coloplast Corporation
www.us.coloplast.com

Medtronic/InterStim® Therapy (Neuromodulation Implant for OAB)
www.medtronic.com
www.bladderdevice.com

General Health and Wellness

Center for Science in the Public Interest
www.cspinet.org

Agency for Healthcare Research and Quality
www.ahrq.gov

U. S. Department of Health and Human Services
www.os.dhhs.gov

Medicare and Medicaid
www.cms.hhs.gov

American Medical Association
www.ama–assn.org

Center for Disease Control and Prevention
www.cdc.gov

U. S. Food and Drug Administration (FDA)
www.fda.gov

{ About the Authors }

— Raymond A. Bologna, M. D. —

Dr. Bologna, a graduate of the University of Notre Dame, received his doctor of medicine from Northeastern Ohio Universities College of Medicine (NEOUCOM) and completed his residency in urology at NEOUCOM's affiliated Urology Program. He went on to complete a fellowship in female pelvic medicine and reconstructive surgery at Graduate Hospital in Philadelphia, Pennsylvania. He then completed a second fellowship in Advanced Pelvic Floor Surgery at SUMMA Health System, Akron, Ohio. Dr. Bologna is co-chairman of Female Pelvic Medicine at Akron General Medical Center and chairman of that same division for the department of Urology at SUMMA Health System. He is also an assistant professor of urology and director of adult research for the Department of Urology at NEOUCOM. Dr. Bologna practices urology and female pelvic medicine and reconstructive surgery in Akron, Ohio.

— Jennifer Heisel Mangano, M. A., P. T. —

Ms. Heisel Mangano received a bachelor of science from The Ohio State University's Physical Therapy Program. She holds a master's degree in exercise physiology from Kent State University, Kent, Ohio. Ms. Heisel Mangano, who specializes in women's health physical therapy, is coordinator of the Women's Health Division of Portage Physical Therapists. She has published a number of articles in her area of specialization and lectures widely on the subject before university, community, and professional audiences.

— J. J. Rodgers —

A long-time writer and editor in the field of health-care marketing and communication, Mr. Rodgers is a graduate of the University of Pennsylvania and holds a master of management from the J. L. Kellogg Graduate School of Management of Northwestern University. His experience includes work in both the pharmaceutical and health insurance industries.

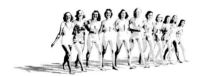

NOTES

NOTES